JOANNA ELLINGTON

Dr. Joanna Ellington ("Dr. E") is an internationally recognized scientist in the area of sexual medicine and sperm physiology with over 75 publications. Her research and expertise have been the topic of several national news stories, including features aired on National Public Radio and published in USA Today. She was a highlighted expert in the television documentaries The Great Sperm Race and Sizing Up Sperm.

Dr. E received her Doctor of Veterinary Medicine from the University of Tennessee in 1984 and a 1990 PhD from Cornell University in the field of reproductive physiology. As an andrologist (a scientist who studies male sexuality and reproduction), her primary area of research has been evaluating the interactions of sperm with the female's Fallopian tube cells while the sperm wait to fertilize an egg. This research led her to invent Pre-Seed®, the world's first fertility-friendly lubricant for couples trying to conceive a child.

She has received numerous grants from the National Institutes of Health and the United States Department of Agriculture, including a prestigious Physician Scientist Award and a First Independent Research in Science Training Award. The scientific community has honored Dr. E's research in sperm physiology with the international Young Andrologist Award. She has also received the Distinguished Alumni Award from the University of Tennessee.

Dr. E reviews and summarizes the latest science on sex, reproduction and intimacy at her website *SexScienceandNature.com*. She has been a featured blogger at *BlogHer.com* and a guest contributor to Cosmopolitan magazine.

Joanna and her husband, Gil, have raised five boys and numerous other critters on their Eastern Washington ranch.

Author's Note

This is a book about the science of sex and how this body of research can lead us to more sexual self-knowledge and fulfillment. In helping to explain what we know about the sexuality of human beings, I have chosen to use the story of my own journey as a woman, from puberty through menopause, as illustration and example. In sections discussing my own life experiences, I have at times changed the names of organizations, people and places. Any similarity between these fictional names and characters in this book and those of real people or entities is strictly a coincidence.

The information written in this book, including sexual and hormonal advice, is the result of my personal experiences and includes my opinions about and interpretations of published studies and other sources. Some of the information, advice and discussions have not been reviewed by the FDA and therefore should not be relied upon to diagnose, treat or cure any condition or disease. Always seek the advice of a physician for a diagnostic and therapeutic plan. As the author, I accept no liability for the reader's use of the information in this book.

Acknowledgments

This book would not have happened without many people believing in it and encouraging me each step of the way. Ryan and Karleen Clifton created the first mock-up of a book "Conceiving Pre-Seed" as a Christmas gift several years ago to remind me of the book waiting to be written. Tyler and Michelle Clifton listened to study after study during family meals as the science for this book came together and also helped remind me that no one is all good or all bad. Casey and Erin Clifton helped us locate the hundreds of studies I reviewed. Our younger boys, Rayne and Sayge, fed the animals and often fended for themselves, even as they had to move stacks of papers about erectile dysfunction or sexually transmitted diseases off the table to eat dinner. Rayne also helped by providing graphics and designs for my Sex, Science and Nature website and social media pages. Sayge continuously reminded me of topics I needed to include in the book, even when I felt "done" with those phases of life. Our grandson Clay never missed an opportunity to try to distract me from my writing, keeping the family/work tension alive throughout this creative process as it has been throughout my adult life.

Amy Gibson provided inspiration and sweat as she dug through thousands of pages of BioOrigyn records to help me remember our amazing journey. She also constantly reaffirmed to me that I had something important to say, even when I wasn't sure. Dr. Jayne Helle helped me to stay focused and patient when I wanted only to be done. She made sure I surrounded this book and everything around it in a warm white light of love, which I hope you will feel. Vicki Meyers-Wallen taught me how to stand up for myself as a woman professionally, as well as how to throw an amazing bachelorette party.

My brothers, sisters, parents and in-laws gave critical insight on different topics, resource support to keep us going when we had nothing left and perspective on human sexuality spanning generations and continents.

Sean Maloney, as always, understood my cover design vision, just as he has for the numerous Pre-Seed cartons and advertisements we have done together throughout the years (including the 2012 Pre-Seed carton that won a national award). Media psychologist and friend Dr. Jenny Fremlin put *SexScienceandNature.com* on the "map" of the internet and gave me the confidence to self publish. Megan Lester and Kathy Arpin carefully edited the book with humor and attention to detail. Dr. Sharon Mortimer helped review literature to find references on some of the more obscure and difficult-to-find topics. Additionally, the ups and downs described in this book couldn't have been navigated without the help of G. Grainger at Washington Trust Bank; Lisa Lester at E2B business services; and our accountants Jim McDirmid and Scott LaPlant.

I am especially grateful to our attorney angels who have believed in, fought for and protected Pre-Seed and our family each step of the way (with many more exciting stories for my next book!). These include Susan Nelson in Spokane; and the folks at Greenberg Traurig Law: Miki Kolton, Claude Wild, Stephen Dietrich and Gayle Strong.

Our friends at First Response™, Fairhaven Health and Earth's Magic have always provided excellent education and products for conception, pregnancy and breastfeeding stages of life. Chris and Suzy DeWolf, and their team at Lil' Drug Store Products, helped Pre-Seed grow and reach even more trying-to-conceive couples.

Michael Gurian, friend and author of *The Wonder of Boys*, read through the more than 600 pages I had written in my attempt to combine the journey of my life with the Pre-Seed adventure and the sexual science I wanted to share with readers. He did a masterful job in helping me narrow down my thoughts to the manageable book you now have, as well as making sure I completed the project!

Finally, I thank my husband, Gilbert Dennis Clifton, the three-in-one: Gil, my cowboy; Dennis, my business partner; and Jack my lover. If there is any doubt, there would be no book without you having done: 1) the cooking, the dishes, the laundry, the animal care and the fence repair; 2) the formatting, the revisions, the reference management and the submission work; and 3) all the things one needs a man to do...such as backing up the horse trailer in a tight spot.

CHARITABLE DONATIONS

At least one percent of all proceeds from this book will be donated to some of my favorite 501c(3) charities. These include:

Work to Ride (*worktoride.net*). This group gives low-income youth the opportunity to interact with horses, including playing the exciting game of polo. I love horses and kids. My favorite is horses, kids, green grass and blue sky – together, having fun. Work to Ride is a community-based prevention program that aids disadvantaged urban youth through activities centered on horsemanship and equine sports. It is a long-term program for 7 to 19 year-old youth who must commit for a minimum of one year (many work throughout high school). Work to Ride graduates receive help with college enrollment. I would like to help this program expand to more cities across the U.S.

La Leche League International (*llli.org*). This group's mission is to "help mothers worldwide to breastfeed through direct mother-to-mother support, encouragement, information and education, and to promote a better understanding of breastfeeding as an important element in the healthy development of the baby and mother." They have other moms waiting to talk to you by phone, in person or online any time you need them. Plus they provide unbiased, scientifically sound reference material to help you make decisions about breastfeeding and childrearing, such as tips for sleeping arrangements, travel and return to work.

"We die containing a richness of lovers and tribes, tastes we have swallowed, bodies we have plunged into and swum up as if rivers of wisdom, characters we have climbed into as if trees, fears we have hidden in as if caves…We are communal histories, communal books. We are not owned or monogamous in our taste or experience."

Michael Ondaatje, *The English Patient*

Table of Contents

Introduction

Everything Is Perfect

"Everything is perfect," said my youngest son's mentor, Tim Corcoran, as the setting sun bathed the Selkirk Mountains in a fiery glow. Reassuringly, this leader of Twin Eagle's Wilderness School repeated the phrase to us, a small group of parents watching our teenage sons walk across a stream into the woods. Our boys were crossing this stream as part of their Rite of Passage as they symbolically left their boyhoods behind. I whispered to myself, "Everything is perfect." As a hawk circled above, I studied the back of my son's head wrapped in a dark blue bandanna, seeing the obvious broad shoulders and narrow hips of a 16-year-old "man." My job of parenting children was done. I would always be a mother but never again a mother to a child. As I stood with my husband, my son's stepfather, I thought, "I have not been a perfect Mom, but in spite of and because of that, everything at this moment is indeed perfect." For two decades, I had cherished doing my part to raise each of our five boys. I had admired each boy through the transition from boyhood to manhood, enjoyed the changing voice, the shifting shape, the sudden burst of sinuous muscles, as well as being one of only a handful of women who (most of the time) still made sense in their rapidly changing lives. I thought again of how grateful I am to have had boys and to have understood the biology and physiology of their maleness with an insight that few people are blessed to have.

I am a female reproductive physiologist who studies men; specifically, I am an andrologist (one who studies "the science of men"). In addition I am a woman and a feminist who admires men. They are not perfect, but in general they are straightforward, transparent, quick to forgive and much less emotionally complex than women. I love many women too, but something about men drew me on a path early in my career to study the science of their sexuality and reproduction, and how they relate to others in intimacy.

Some of you may know me as "Dr. E" from my work studying sperm or helping infertile couples and from my website Sex, Science and Nature. You may have seen me in the TV documentaries The Great Sperm Race and National Geographic's Sizing Up Sperm or heard me on National Public Radio talking about my research and my pet pig. As a scientist (beginning as a veterinarian and then moving to human science), I have spent thirty years studying sexuality and reproduction. My USDA and National Institutes of Health funded research focused on how the female's Fallopian tube cells select and nurture the best sperm so they can reach and fertilize the egg. In this research, I learned that human conception is not the "battle" between sexes it is often portrayed to be, but rather, it is an intricately timed collaboration between the male and female in their quest to create new life.

Research into this process would have been enough to satisfy me professionally had I not stumbled onto something completely unexpected. That something was Pre-Seed®, the world's first "fertility" lubricant, which has had a profound impact on people's lives in ways I could never have imagined. I discovered Pre-Seed by chance. Initially, during my federally funded research, I learned that many trying-to-conceive (TTC) couples were using "nonspermicidal" lubricants to make "having-to-have sex" to conceive a baby more comfortable and fun, without knowing that these products may harm sperm. During this research I, like many other scientists who have made remarkable discoveries, had an experiment that "failed," resulting in the serendipitous discovery of a natural plant sugar, arabinogalactan, which offers antioxidant protection and support for sperm.

After this finding, I teamed with colleagues to develop Pre-Seed as a lubricant that instead of harming sperm, actually provides sperm with an optimal environment for their journey to the egg. Since its launch in 2003, Pre-Seed has sold millions of doses around the world, and we have received thousands of deeply moving stories from users and physicians alike regarding Pre-Seed's beneficial impact on people's lives. When sex works as it should, when it is comfortable and fun and the sperm finds its journey "slippery when wet," people often conceive! And even beyond sex for conception, Pre-Seed's mild isotonic (balanced salt) formulation has been called in independent studies one of the safest water-soluble lubricants for its gentleness and lack of irritation. This is important because many everyday lubricants can cause tissue damage and may even increase sexually transmitted infection (STI) rates.

Between my scientific studies and developing and bringing this unique product to the retail shelf, I have learned a great deal about human sexuality and intimacy. But in addition to having spent my career working in sexual science, I am also just like "every woman" who makes her way through life, sex, and intimacy. Each of us feels empowered at times and ridiculous at others as we move into and out of our confident sexual selves. In my case, I can talk about reproduction on national TV but am deeply embarrassed to buy "personal items" at the store (I always try to bury them under other items in my cart, even adding things I don't need just to cover them up). And while doing my scientific work, I have been a wife, mother and sexual partner, navigating prolonged and significant health issues and the emotional stress of attempted hostile company takeovers, as well as divorce, remarriage and blended families.

My science is thus my life, and I am eager to share with you some of what I have learned about sex and intimacy as a scientist, as a woman and as an andrologist. I hope that learning more about the science of sex will give you a renewed sense of power about who you are sexually, as well as an understanding that we are all pretty normal, even within a variety of sexual expressions. I also hope to reassure you that having sexual issues, of all shapes and sizes, is part and parcel of the human experience, and that with science and understanding we can all navigate these times, just as I have had to do.

Through my own sexual journey, I've learned that I am a lot stronger than I thought I could be. I also realize that every person and couple must find their own internal rhythms and a deeper sexual self-knowledge if women and men (and women and women and men and men) are going to find happiness, peace and joy in their intimacy. As we'll explore together in this book, sex is that important. Much of marriage and successful life actually depends on how we feel about our sex lives, even when we don't realize it. Ultimately, I have written this book with the hope that my personal story matched with scientific knowledge will help you, whatever your age, to enjoy the science of sex and the pleasure of love in exciting new ways. I will also offer some new items for your sexual "toolbox" which I hope may give you greater confidence to enhance your own sexual fulfillment.

Occasionally, you will also find my **Radical Center Ruminations,** where I would ask you to stop and think about how as a society we can encourage public and private conversation on controversial topics beyond our current never-ending stale battles around sex. We don't need unreasonable moral polarizations any more—we need a Radical Center in which to stand together and honestly confront aspects of our evolving sexuality. If as a society we can start thinking and talking about these topics, we can better move forward in creating the healthy sexuality we want and need.

One Woman's Sexual Story

Because sexuality is so intimately a part of a person's unique self, it is difficult to speak of it with credibility and accuracy from just a cold, scientific viewpoint. Thus, this book weaves my own sexual story with the scientific work from my research and that of others. As you read this book, if you find that I reveal or prescribe something offensive to you, I hope that you'll see the greater context of my exploration and forgive my offenses enough to keep reading. My wish in sharing my story is for every one of us to find a future where sexual science provides the knowledge we need to better connect with others, as well as to empower ourselves sexually, however we choose for that to manifest itself.

Why Being 'Slippery When Wet' Matters

Before we begin this journey together, I thought I would share some of my favorite real-life stories from people about their experiences with the lubricant I developed. I have specifically chosen these comments because they show how sex impacts life on so many different levels—from the sheer, intimate ecstasy of great lovemaking, to the importance of conceiving our children, to the process of regaining a woman's femininity after battling cancer. These stories illustrate that everyone can build a more fulfilling sex life through a better understanding of sexual science and a willingness to seek solutions. These words also give you a window into my world and the joy my work has given me over the past decade. Thank you for joining with me as we turn the page and start looking at the mystery of sex together in exciting, new ways.

Sex is fun, not painful anymore

"Oh My Goodness...I got my Pre-Seed in the mail yesterday... Then ran back upstairs. Read instructions... Proceeded to begin baby dance (intercourse)... It was Amazing! It didn't hurt to have sex! I'd say 90% of the time I am trying to not focus on some level of pain, while trying to relax and enjoy... And when I used other products like KY it just felt weird. Messy, think, un-natural feeling, and it didn't really do much for the pain. But today...today probably for the first time in a long time, if ever, I made love to my husband and I was there in the moment not focusing on pain, because it wasn't there. No pain just pleasure. I cried to know that sex can feel good...!"

Seven years of frustration are over

"My wife and I tried to conceive for seven (yes seven!) years and spent over $35,000 at a fertility clinic, with no results... We just accepted that we may never be able to conceive... One evening almost two years ago, a news anchor mentioned how some people were successfully conceiving using some sort of kit. I went upstairs, logged on to the Internet and began my research... I soon came across your product and ordered Pre-Seed. Honestly, we were happy to have found another method that was very low stress, natural, and relatively inexpensive, but I don't think we truly believed it would work...but it did work after only three months of trying. I will NEVER forget coming home to my wife waiting at the door with a little plastic thing that said "Pregnant"! Nothing had even said this once in seven years, and there it was. She started crying and I did too... The delivery of our son went as close to perfectly as one could hope... Thank you so much for your incredible product..."

Learning to feel pleasure again after cancer

"When it came to intimacy with my partner after my cancer treatment was finished, lubrication wasn't a problem - but my pelvic floor muscles were too tight to allow intercourse. This was a reaction of my body to the pelvic cancer, and so I needed to go through a course of physical therapy to "retrain" my pelvic floor to allow penetration during lovemaking. Part of this physical therapy required the use of vaginal dilators to stretch "my parts" back out. I used Pre-Seed to lubricate the dilators during the physical therapy. I loved that the Pre-Seed felt like "natural" lubrication, which made a very clinical process much more relaxing, leading to a successful outcome. Thank you for helping me find joy in being intimate again!"

Chapter 1

Just Like Animals

I grew up "down on the farm," in a life filled with animals of all shapes and sizes, complete with both the joys and the messes this resulted in. As the eldest daughter of a full-time preacher and a "preacher's wife" (which likewise is a full-time job), I was also privy to the messiness of human life. The local pastor is there to celebrate human relationships that succeed and to pick up the pieces for those that fail. They stand side by side with people from all classes and walks of life during the hardest of times: addictions, sudden illness, infidelity, unplanned pregnancies, murder and suicide. Pastors are the support of last resort. Growing up at our house meant understanding the complexity and consequences of human intimacy in a way few people experience.

In contrast, the animals on our farm often provided blessedly straightforward interactions. They wanted clean water and food (on time!) and to have sex, reproduce and care for their young. Seeing mating and birthing animals was a routine, natural part of life. I also saw death—both acceptable, for meat to feed our family, and tragic, when someone forgot to feed or water their animals or when gates were left open. I learned early on to finish what I started and to care for the vulnerable among us.

By the time I reached fifth grade, the one animal we didn't have on our farm was a horse, but I knew my parents didn't have the money to buy one. So I decided to earn the funds myself. To this end, I handwrote index cards offering my services as a housekeeper, and at ten years of age dropped off the cards in mailboxes of homes around us. Several women took me up on the offer, and I started working six hours a week cleaning homes at one dollar an hour. Each week, I put my earnings into an old cigar box covered in purple pen tally marks to keep track of my financial progress. Finally, on Christmas day I received a large boost in the form of a twenty-dollar bill from my parents and five dollars from my Granny. In the local paper I saw an ad for a Saddlebred mare for $125, the exact amount I had in my box! Dad drove us out to a neighboring farm where we found a Chestnut mare, Sandy, with a flaxen mane and tail, and a mean temperament. She had just broken her owner's nose by tossing her head in anger during a ride.

"Be careful. And always tie her head down," the owner warned us.

Dad wanted me to think twice about buying her, but she was the only horse I could afford. When you are an eleven-year-old girl, there is no such thing as a bad horse. And I never once tied Sandy's head down after we brought her home. In fact, Sandy turned out not only to be my first horse, but also to be a kind of mirror for me—independent, a bit of a troublemaker and always ready to go.

Sadly, several years after I bought her, she died from tetanus. At that time, my family knew nothing about vaccines or basic horse care other than to worm them and make sure they had plenty to eat and drink, so Sandy was not protected by the necessary annual horse vaccines. Tetanus causes a slow, agonizing death. My close friend, Anna, and I stayed up for forty-eight hours singing every song we knew to Sandy. When it was finally hopeless, and the vet came to put her down, I knew then and there that being a veterinarian was part of what I wanted to do with my life. I wanted to be able to keep animals from having to go through what Sandy and I had experienced. I didn't realize at the time that the natural flow of farm life would eventually lead me even more specifically into the specialized study of sex and reproduction.

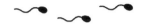

Growing up as a preacher's kid (a "PK") and a farm hand, I felt the visceral duality people have around sex. On the one hand, sex and the relationship between the male and female members of a species were day-to-day business in the barnyard. The rooster chased the hen for a quick roll in the dirt, but as Granny (who lived to be 107 years old) would say, "Did the little red hen run as fast as she can?" implying that the hen really wanted to get caught. On the farm, sex was sex, with a hint of both surrender and whimsical adventure to it. But on the other hand, being the daughter of a prominent pastor and very much in the public eye, my behavior as I matured was often fodder for judgment, constant comment and shaming, in a way that didn't mesh with the practicality of what I saw on the farm. It seemed odd to me that something as natural as sex and reproduction in animals changed for humans, where it became chaotic and complicated. I, like most young people, felt unsure of what being sexual would mean for me as an adult.

What is Normal Sex?

Each of us, in early adolescence and on into our adulthood, asks ourself this question many times. Scientists answer this by looking for *baselines* for the sexual activities they are studying in a population. These are the everyday occurrences of intimacy, the "what we do, when and how often" of lovemaking and sex. To begin our exploration into the science of sexuality, think about your own "sexual baseline." It may be one that is very expansive (i.e., including a lot of sexual partners, experiences, positions and experiments) or it could be limited to just you knowing your own body and its responses. Whatever your baseline, it is yours, and for all of us these sexual baselines bring both beauty and limitation. As you ponder your own history, check out the sexual baseline data from recent national surveys. Let's see what we can learn about sexual "normalcy" in our culture. Figures adapted from Herbenick and colleagues, 2010 and Reece and colleagues, 2010.

Figure 1. Percentage of Americans engaging in solo masturbation in the last 90 days by gender and relationship status (single or married).

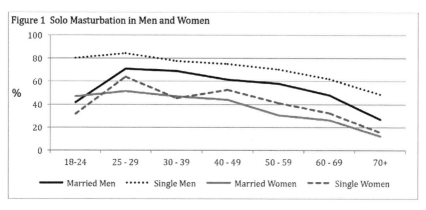

Figure 2. Percentage of Americans engaging in different sexual practices in the past 90 days for: a) Married Women; b) Married Men; c) Single Women; and d) Single Men.

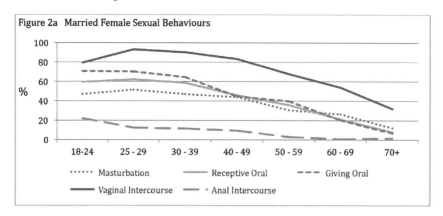

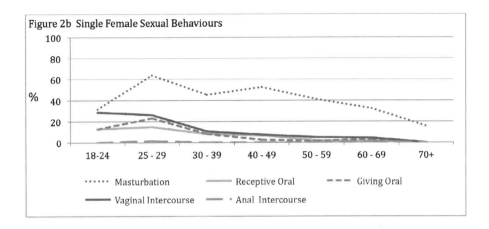

Figure 2b Single Female Sexual Behaviours

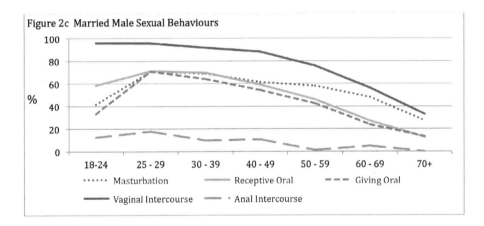

Figure 2c Married Male Sexual Behaviours

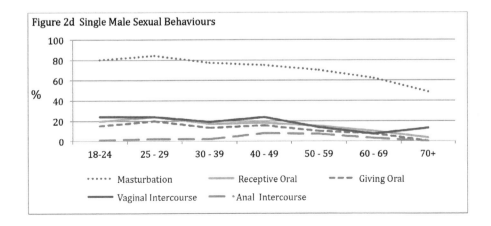

Figure 2d Single Male Sexual Behaviours

Solo Masturbation Is Commonplace, Even Among Married People

Many of us masturbate, even if we are married. While we may each know this personally because we have masturbated recently, we might not realize that so has just about everyone else! In fact masturbation is part of many people's sexual baseline, and it can be our first sex act. Here are a few facts about masturbation in America.

- Close to half of women and three quarters of men have masturbated by themselves in the past 90 days.

- Being married doesn't decrease masturbation rates all that much, especially for women.

- Masturbation is the most common sexual activity for men, with over 30% through age 40 doing it more than twice a week. In contrast, most women masturbate several times a month rather than weekly.

- Although a decline in masturbation activities occurs with age, even at age 70, around 20% of women and 40% of men remain active.

- Masturbation remains an important part of single people's sex lives, with four times more single people having masturbated in the past 90 days than single people having had partnered intercourse in that same time frame.

Hopefully, knowing that most other people masturbate can help us sense the normalcy of it. If you are in a couple, you can measure your sexual maturity with one another by whether you can discuss masturbation freely, with humor and a sense of experimentation.

And ladies, don't take it personally if he masturbates alone sometimes (just like many of you girls). Masturbation is most likely a part of his sexual baseline and has been since long before you met him. An occasional whank in the shower or when no one else is home is perfectly fine. And at times masturbation is necessary for everyone's sanity, such as after the birth of a child or if a partner is ill—when one of you isn't getting much sex with the other. However, if things are not going well sexually for your partnership, you may need to say to your partner, "I am having to turn to masturbation more than I want to, and we need to talk about why this is happening." Since some masturbation in marriage may be due to poor quality sex for the woman (she isn't reaching orgasm with him, for instance) or not enough sex for the man, we often push these discussions aside—as we want to avoid the sexual conflict. Because all marriages go through phases of more and less sexual activity, it isn't necessarily bad to just let things go for a while. However, if "the sex talk" is not happening after three or more months of a changed sexual baseline (meaning too much masturbation and not enough partnered sex), it is generally important to talk about what's going on.

A good indication that it's time for the talk is if either of you feel you are using masturbation as a replacement for sex with your partner because it is easier and less hassle than initiating or having sex. If you are feeling the loss of a healthy sexual baseline in your relationship, your partner will also likely be feeling something is wrong. In fact, in a recent study, both men and women accurately perceived their partner's level of sexual satisfaction at a much higher rate than previously anticipated by sex scientists. If one of you feels a lack in your sex life and is filling that space with masturbation, you both realize this at some level. You need to talk about it.

Sex Varies in Its Expression

From the graphs shown, you can see that many forms of sexual expression are normal for human beings. We are sexual creatures, and we are sexually exploratory. That said, the basic staple of married sex is still penile-vaginal intercourse (PVI), whether missionary position, doggie-style or another. The next most popular sex is giving and receiving oral sex, then partnered masturbation, and lastly anal intercourse. As we age, our rate of PVI steadily declines; however, 50% of married men and women into their 60s and 30% into their 70s still remain active in this way. And these rates will likely continue to increase as aging men and women grow in comfort with taking Hormone Replacement Therapy (HRT). Interestingly, married women between the ages of 18 to 24 have less vaginal intercourse than many other groups, maybe because they are giving 30% more unreciprocated oral sex to their men! Or maybe it is just as a means of avoiding pregnancy.

Receiving and giving oral sex is a normal part of our marriages, with over half of couples into their 40s sharing this form of intimacy, and most giving as good as they get. Partnered masturbation becomes especially important to the sexual baselines of aging adults as a partner experiences poor health (it is used twice as much in these couples as compared to age-matched couples with excellent health).

Anal sex happens relatively infrequently (with less than 15% of married men and women having had it recently), but it is still part of a normal sexual baseline for human beings. Anal finger play and rimming (licking) are much more common than anal intercourse, occurring at more than twice the rate of anal intercourse.

Interestingly, men who are dating receive the most oral sex of any group, with 81% recently enjoying this form of intimacy. In recent studies, over 60% of women, ages 25 to 39 who were single and dating used partnered masturbation in their sex lives, in some part because it is safest for avoiding sexually transmitted infections and unwanted pregnancies.

Although over half of single women in their 30s and 40s continue to regularly masturbate, the percentage of these women engaging in partnered sexual activity dramatically declines. This can be a source of joy for some women and great sadness or loneliness for others. The scientists who do this valuable work to track our sexual baselines, such as Dr. Debby Herbenick, also have written excellent, entertaining and easy to read resource books to help improve solo and partnered sex for women, such as *Because It Feels Good: A Woman's Guide to Sexual Pleasure and Satisfaction* and *Read My Lips: A Complete Guide to the Vagina and Vulva*. If you are a single man or woman, know that you deserve great sex too. Don't be shy about buying toys, candles and warming oils for special times for yourself. It doesn't make you "weird"— it makes you sensual! Dr. Castellanos, "The Sex MD," recommends in *How to Get Over 5 Internal Roadblocks to Good Sex* that all adults orgasm at least once or twice a week (either through sex or masturbation), to best preserve the function of our sexual organs. Retaining your sensuality, for yourself or to share with someone else later, is an important part of staying happy and healthy.

Aging and Sexuality

Although some folks are happy to let their sexual identity fade into the sunset, others will fight with every prescription known to man to protect and preserve theirs (count me in here!). Therefore, no particular age group is without its sexual baseline. In a recent study of people in their 80s, around 20% of women and 40% of men reported engaging in sex or masturbation in the past year. The most common reasons cited for not being sexually active was lack of desire (for women) and erectile dysfunction (for men). When sexually inactive seniors were asked if they would like to resume having sex, 35% of women and 85% of men said, "Yes." However, only 10% of senior women and 30% of senior men had ever discussed the topic with their physician. In fact, 70% of older women report that sexual health was never brought up during their routine annual physical exam, in spite of the fact that sexually transmitted disease infection rates are growing among senior citizens.

It is essential that everyone over fifty initiates discussions about their sexual concerns and goals with their doctors. Remember that your doctor isn't bringing these up to you because he or she may not want to offend you. But these providers can help optimize your sex life. Having sex is one of the healthiest forms of exercise and intimacy that seniors can engage in—it can even increase your lifespan! So go for it as and when you can and get help to enhance your sex life if needed. It is also okay to discuss what you need to protect yourself and to optimize your sexuality even if you aren't in a relationship and you are just hoping to "get lucky," like my neighbor in her weekly bowling group. After a year of enjoying her bowling "occasional hookup guy," these two wild ones married in their late 70s and are now in the happiest time of their lives!

Radical Center Ruminations - How, where and when should seniors have sex? Maybe there should be special "hotel room" suites that seniors can schedule within their assisted living facility. Privacy for sexual expression shouldn't be a class-based right (e.g., only for those who can afford a private room). When does dementia preclude someone from having the right to sexual consent? Institutionalized patients (for any number of reasons, including Alzheimers) with spouses at home may choose to have extramarital sex. Should the facility staff intervene and tell the other partner or not? Should facilities be able to restrict gay or bisexual senior sex based on religious beliefs? Sexually transmitted diseases are on the rise in Baby Boomers. Seniors themselves, as well as housing and socialization centers for this group, need to be honest about this natural and exciting part of senior life. Bring senior sex out of the "grey closet"!

The Tale of Two Sisters

Sexual baselines can vary dramatically for people. When I was young, I was exposed through two great aunts to two very different views of sexuality. At one extreme, Aunt Lily referred to sex as "that terrible thing" she had to do "once a month." Both Aunt Lily and her husband were vibrant, physically active people well into their 80s, but sex was never mentioned and certainly not ever joked about in their home. In contrast, Aunt Jean and her horse trainer husband had sex nearly every day of their married lives until he was killed in a riding accident at 63. Even when Jean was in her 80s and suffering from dementia, she loved nothing more than to talk about her favorite positions for sex and how she and her husband would sneak away for quickies in the barn. When I was young, I wasn't quite sure how people ended up with such divergent views on the role of sex in their lives. Now I know that even I, a sexually active woman, couldn't keep up with Aunt Jean! And I feel sad for Aunt Lily and her husband. Something that could and should have provided them with joy wasn't nurtured correctly and never fully blossomed between them. Perhaps they were never given the science to fully understand their sexual selves and how to develop healthy baselines, starting with their developing sexuality during adolescence.

Chapter 2

Teen Times

For me, adolescence was an awkward time. I was a unique teenager, dressing in hats with veils, or braiding my hair with flowers and wrapping this long, flower-filled hair around my neck like a scarf (granted it was the 70s). Because I have a difficult name to pronounce correctly, Joanna…pronounced like "Joanna, marijuana" or "Joanna, do you wanna," I started going by Joe—with just that masculine spelling—so that I could avoid the name teasing and express my tomboy nature.

All this might have seemed to set me up to be an outcast, but I was longtime friends with the then popular girls so I circulated on the edges of the "cool" kids. Although I was always among the last to be asked to go to Homecoming or other big dances, this didn't stop me from developing friends with (limited) benefits. Many weekends I would end up "parking" in the high school lot during basketball games with some guy or another from our group. Not much happened beyond second base as we groped and kissed in the front seat of someone's car, but when I would return to the gym, I would inevitably receive an outraged lecture from my friends who scolded me for not behaving the way a "Preacher's Kid" should behave. "The boys are using you!" they insisted, but to me the making out and touching felt more like mutual "usury" since neither I nor the guys felt much passion for one another. Experimentation and learning were my motives, not true love.

During my senior year of high school, my parents moved back east, but I stayed in our hometown to graduate, living in the basement of family friends, working twenty hours a week to support myself. This change made the high school censorship even worse as my friends believed they needed to look out for me while my parents were gone. One night before graduation, I made it to a friend's house late after work for a party. When I arrived, I saw that everyone was completely drunk. Kevin, the most popular guy in our class, lay passed out behind the couch, against the wall. Worried for him, I knelt down to talk to him and see if he needed help. By the time I had given him a pillow and finally just decided to let him sleep it off, fifteen minutes had passed. I thought nothing of this encounter as I gave other people rides and headed home for a shower and bed.

On the following Monday at school (this was before cell phones and Facebook), no one would talk to me, not even my best friends. Even now I can recall my uncertainty and anxiety trying to figure out what I had done to cause this shunning. Finally, a close friend told me that she was furious that I had been "making out" with Kevin behind the couch. Her anger and that of the whole school shocked me. Kevin didn't have a girlfriend, so I remember thinking at the time, "Yeah, what if I had been?" But instead of voicing my feelings, I reassured her and everyone else that "Nothing happened!" while feeling internally furious that these girls who had boyfriends and active sex lives felt such authority to judge and dictate who I should be. As adversity often does, this event led me to adopt one of the guiding principles of my life: living to please other people is a thankless, zero sum game. Few things are worse than people without full, active lives, plotting away and telling us how to manage our lives.

A Scientist's Guidebook for Sex Ed in Teens

Thinking back to my own adolescence has been very useful to me, not only professionally, but as I have raised our five boys. Our boys include three stepsons from my husband, Gil, and my two biological sons. The boys cover a twelve-year age gap, and all entered into our blended family during high school or younger. For these boys, growing up with parents who made and sold Pre-Seed, a sex lubricant, was a source of both pride and embarrassment. I remember an elementary Open House when our son Rayne (#4 in our age order of boys) made a drawing of a sperm cell fertilizing an egg and explained that his mom helped "make babies." In another incident, soon after Gil and I married, our son Tyler (#3) sighed, "Do we have to talk about sperm at dinner again tonight?" And of course there was the slide photo at one of our boy's high school graduations showing a senior girl's car covered in 5 gallons of Pre-Seed and wrapped in Saran Wrap®. The students all howled when the photo came on the screen, the parents looked confused, and I sank down in my seat just a bit…but it was pretty funny!

Over the years, how I talk with all our boys about sex, especially during their adolescence, has evolved. I've made some errors and felt many of the frustrations you may have felt. My credo has always been this: engage with our kids about sex as much as possible, in an age-appropriate manner (aware that "appropriate" is unique for each child's own maturation pace). Human adolescence today holds unique challenges. While in the past adolescents had sex for the purpose of procreation and pleasure, our adolescents are either having some form of sex solely for pleasure and experimentation, or are exposed to nonstop sexual content through electronic media in ways unheard of in our human past. I have found that the best parenting involves connection and communication, teaching and mentoring, listening and being there.

Many people worry that discussing sex with our kids will prod them to "do it," but if you are one of these people, please know that there is no scientific evidence to support this fear. In fact, just the opposite is true. Helping adolescents feel empowered and knowledgeable about the physiology and emotionality of intimacy and giving them a safe place to discuss anything and everything that is happening around them allows kids to better manage the pressure to have sex they feel from both friends and dating partners.

Here's an example from my own family. One of our boys at 16 came to me obviously agitated after a New Year's Eve party. "Mom, Kylie told me she could light fireworks in my pants last night. I know I'm not ready to have sex, but she is really pushing me." After doing an internal end zone victory dance that my son knew he didn't want to take this step, I asked him what he liked about Kylie and what they had in common. When nothing about working with animals or being outdoors came up, I asked him about these two topics (they were and are his deep life-loves). He replied, "She gets nervous being outside." I calmly but emphatically reminded him that absolutely everyone he has sex with is a potential co-parent with him for life. I stressed that his life would be profoundly difficult and sad if he had to co-parent a child with a mother who did not share his sense of connectivity with the natural world. The next day he told Kylie he was "too busy" to continue seeing her (Yes!).

Radical Center Ruminations - Recently I tried to get my youngest son's health records for a school physical, only to be told that because he is over 14 years old, I (his mom) can't access the records without his permission. I understand the logic—the state wants to protect children's rights to birth control and reproductive health (the law is trying to protect my son)—but, to me, this also keeps sex too secret, too behind-closed-doors, and it discards accountability between the teen and parent. In fact, I'm not exactly sure how we parents came to agree with policy-makers that we should relinquish our right to know what our kids are doing at age

14 as if puberty equals self-determination. I don't know about your adolescents, but when my boys were 14, they needed help just keeping track of their lunch boxes. I am not convinced they can or should be left alone to sort out who they are sexually, without parental involvement. In Washington State, where I live, children can't leave home or emancipate themselves until age 16. Shouldn't health care access and health records be jointly available to parent and child until at least 16?

What Teens Today Need to Know

Sex education for my own children has grown from my work as a scientist. I believe that we each need more knowledge about a process or system rather than less and especially about a human function that permeates all aspects of our lives. Let's remember: once puberty hits, kids think about sex or "romance" many times per day and that's just the tip of the iceberg. The iceberg itself involves sex hormones as a primary driving force in the development of the teen's brain chemistry, morality, psychology, sociology, neurology and spirituality. I grew up in a household that was open about the joys of sex within marriage, but there wasn't much room to discuss different sexual approaches to life. I, in partnership with their fathers, have taught my own kids more specifically about the physiology and psychology of sexuality and intimacy relatively early in their lives.

Using the animals around us on our farm, our elementary-age boys understood how sex "works." I have especially thought this is important for boys, so that they can understand how sperm are made and better protect their own reproductive future. When one of our sons was diagnosed with juvenile epilepsy, part of the detailed conversation between our son, the physician and us parents was the potential effect of the medication on puberty and future sperm production. My son was well able to understand and voice his opinion and concerns on this topic at age 11.

When each of our boys turned 16, they received a box of condoms. Yet we also drove home the message that we did not feel that they were ready to have sexual intercourse. We often discussed the fact that their lives were awesome, fun and busy. And that they had a lifetime to have sex with its joys and hassles, and that focusing on something else in high school would allow for a more full life in the long haul. My husband and I also taught the health of masturbation. "You have a right or left hand and all the Pre-Seed lubricant needed in bedrooms and showers…put them to good use."

We also wanted each of our young men to learn about and understand female reproductive anatomy and sexual function. Having hubby preach the importance of the clitoris and female orgasm to our older teens helped emphasize their future roles as partners in creating mutually fulfilling relationships.

Where the Heck Is That Clitoris?

Knowledge about the anatomy and physiology of the clitoris is important education for teens of both sexes. Unfortunately, a lot of young people grow up in ignorance of this complex organ. In a recent study, nineteen-year-old men and women were asked about their understanding of the clitoris. At surprisingly similar rates, 29% of women and 25% of men could not locate the external clitoris on a diagram of the vulva. As my boys were growing up, and when it became appropriate, we made sure they understood what this part of the female body was and did. For the sake of their future partners, I did not want them to be sexually illiterate.

For girls, self-knowledge is critical in order for them to develop healthy sexual identities. This "*Cliteracy*," as coined by Sophia Wallace, can of course help girls learn self-pleasuring. Additionally, this knowledge is valuable for girls and young women because once we have experienced pleasure in our own bodies then we can share these secrets with our partners, helping make sex more fulfilling for both of us.

Many teens, including girls themselves, share confusion about female genitalia, such as not understanding the anatomy of the clitoris or mixing and matching the terms vulva and vagina (because societally we use these terms incorrectly all the time). Additionally most girls aren't taught basic physiology, such as how their bodies lubricate for sex; why overstimulation of the clitoris (by an untaught partner or super tight jeans) can cause pain rather than pleasure; and what will and will not work to trigger an orgasm. Telling our daughters about these things does not make girls promiscuous. The best scientific evidence shows the contrary. By teaching girls about who they are as women, we give them more strength to withstand the sexual pressures of adolescence. By teaching them how to experience self-pleasure, they can discover and develop an internal language for themselves regarding the types of touch, activities and images that make them feel sexually responsive, as well as giving them clarity as to what they don't like sexually.

Throughout human history, nearly all of our ancestors spent a good deal of time both with reproducing animals and in small living spaces where people had sex. Children, from a very young age, learned much more about "real" sex than our children do today because they observed or heard animals, their parents and/or other adults having sex on a routine basis. Thus, the human brain, as is developmentally appropriate, can handle much more information about real-life sex than we realize—we are wired to do so.

Masturbation, a Private or Public Topic?

In 1994, the American Surgeon General, Jocelyn Elders, was forced to resign because of her support for a public discussion of teen masturbation in Sex Ed classes. She argued that masturbation was a means to prevent STIs, HIV and unwanted pregnancies. Politics destroyed her, but her wisdom was scientifically sound. The more kids learn about masturbation, the better off, in general, society and our individual teens will be because for most adolescents, masturbating can be helpful in many ways, including keeping early intercourse at bay.

Most boys don't need to be taught about masturbation; it is something they learn and practice regularly. In fact, I recall a recent camping trip when my husband and the boys (all of them acting like 7th graders) spent fifteen minutes coming up with all the names people use for male masturbation. Wow, the list was long! Our favorite term was "loping the mule." In general, boys teach themselves what turns them on and through this develop an early internal language regarding their sexual functioning.

In contrast, girls often first experience sexual arousal, not by themselves, but rather through physical intimacy with boys, including during intercourse. Because many women do not readily orgasm during penile-vaginal intercourse, girls are much less likely to experience early sexual encounters in which orgasm is a natural conclusion to feeling aroused. Additionally, the number of women for whom their first time of making love feels good is much lower than that found for men. In one study, 36% of men and 10% of women considered their first intercourse *very pleasurable* whereas 5% of men versus 33% of women found it very *unpleasant*. Many girls feel embarrassed to admit that they didn't enjoy sex and unsure what they can do to improve their fulfillment and reach orgasm. I know some parents are reading this and thinking, "Good, then she won't do it again!" But if your daughter has already had bad sex, the chance that she won't keep having sex is very small. And coming to accept herself as a woman who "just doesn't respond" can saddle her with years of failed relationships and poor self-esteem.

Fostering a relationship where girls can talk about their own sexual concerns and disappointments with a parent or other trusted adult can help raise her expectations and allow her to be more assertive and selective in the future. A little openness can go a long way in limiting actual numbers of lifetime sexual partners. It can also help our girls feel more at ease in self-discovery, as well as giving them an understanding that sex isn't something that "happens to them." Just like any physical activity it is an exercise they can, and hopefully will, learn to get better and better at, even if they decide to wait before learning more.

Overall, orgasms are healthy for the human body and brain, whether a person is a teen or a senior citizen. As is developmentally appropriate for each adolescent, we as parents and mentors ought to encourage the kind of self-discovery that orgasm leads to, rather than curtail it. Research shows that women with a history of masturbation and orgasmic response in activities other than penile-vaginal intercourse feel significantly more deserving of sexual pleasure and better able to achieve such enjoyment during their adult years. This female sexual pleasure is a common denominator in healthy and happy marriages.

The Sexual Activity of American Youth

In Chapter 1, we identified the "sexual baseline" for adults; now let's look at this for American teens. A recent national survey reviewed data from 15 to 24-year-old women and found the average age of first sexual intercourse was 16, with 36% of girls having their first intercourse at 15 years of age or less. Lifetime sexual experiences for these young women included: penile-vaginal intercourse (64%); oral sex (64%); and anal sex (20%). Half of the young women had one sexual partner, *but a quarter had six or more partners by 24 years of age.* Eight percent reported a sexually transmitted infection, although this low incidence suggests that some girls may have had sexually transmitted diseases and not realized or reported it. Close to 20% reported ever being pregnant. Interestingly, while having had vaginal sex in the past 90 days has been found to correlate with good health in 18 to 25-year-old women, for the younger girls in this study (as young as 15) all forms of sexual intimacy were correlated with lower health quality.

This negative relationship between sex and health for girls under 18 may be because of the link between sexual behavior in adolescents and depression. Many of these sexually active girls are feeling pressured into unfulfilling sex and intimacy at a time that our society is split between messages that "all sex should be great sex" and "all sex (in teens) is bad sex." Often, young women (and some young men) end up having "compliant" sex. "Compliant sex" means they really don't want to go forward with it, but they have intercourse in order to:

- Gain sexual experience (51% males versus 34% females)

- Give in to peer pressure (31% vs 16%)

- Gain popularity (12% vs 6%)

- Ensure a partner won't leave (17% vs 32%)

- Increase the probability of a long-term relationship (9% vs 44%)

These last two points are tricky. On average, adolescent girls typically feel greater love and commitment after sexual union than adolescent boys. Males, in contrast, are more likely to view a partner as less attractive and sexy a few hours after intercourse. Much of this is due to the chemistry of testosterone and oxytocin in bloodstreams after orgasm. This finding is especially true for young men with high numbers of past sex partners. Thus, one message we can give young women and gay teens, if we want to help them put off their first intercourse, is to let them know that research shows "putting out" (compliant sex) doesn't usually work to get the guy. It also isn't a successful strategy for keeping a man. Allowing unwanted intercourse in order to avoid conflict with a partner (so the partner won't become angry or withdraw) also doesn't work. Unfortunately, this type of "avoidance sex" (when someone has sex to avoid losing the partner's affection) actually leads to more lifetime risky sexual behaviors, more lifetime partners, more STIs, less effective birth control and more unplanned pregnancy.

Radical Center Ruminations - Let's teach correct anatomy, physiology and function in our Sex Ed classes, especially that of the woman. Every high school student should know the difference between the vulva and the vagina. For a great read for parents, educators and teens, check out Dr. Castellano's work "Stop Saying Vagina Unless You Mean It" (*SexMD.com*). Teens should also know the true anatomy of the clitoris and arousal tissues in women; how natural lubrication occurs; and the cervical mucus secretion patterns that indicate a woman's fertile times of the month. Additionally, masturbation for both sexes should be discussed as the fact of life that it is, specifically that it is normal and common as a means to sexual self-knowledge and to delay partnered sexual activity. Taboos existing in culture and religion can also be mentioned, and kids should be encouraged to know their own culture or family stance on the topic. Talking in a healthy way at home and at school about sex and different attitudes towards intimacy helps our teens develop language around sexuality that can actually strengthen their ability to say "no."

Social Negotiations and Sex

In high school I had a short fling with Dash, a tall, muscular, Hawaiian football player. Dash wasn't in my normal friendship group and didn't know my family, so there was no pressure on how I "should act." In fact, the pressure from Dash was the opposite. He was interested in dating a "Haole" (a white girl) because his friends were getting the action they wanted from us mainland girls. Dash and I had fun going to the drive-in movies or for long walks at night on the shores of Lake Washington (in Seattle) where he taught me how to handle his "equipment." Meanwhile, I remained adamant that I didn't want to have intercourse with him. Finally, after a month of enjoying each other's company, he told me he would not continue to see me if I wouldn't have sex with him. As much as I enjoyed not being with someone from our insular group at school, I knew this wasn't a place I wanted to go. In the end I was happy to have developed the inner compass from my upbringing to negotiate saying no when I didn't want to become sexually active yet—even though it meant the end of a relationship.

Communication skills and sex may not seem that related, but for young people, the ability to develop "social negotiation skills" is a strong predictor of whether or not an individual will engage in risky sexual behavior (such as not having a partner use a condom or having multiple partners). I explained social negotiation skills to our boys this way: "Can you stop a course of action you don't really want to do (such as having sex with the drunk girl your buddies are pushing you towards) and do it in a way that doesn't harm your friendships with these people?" These are tough things to do for adolescent boys—and even tougher for girls. Girls often feel they "owe" sex if a male is aroused. In fact, 63% of teens view the male sex drive as "uncontrollable," and 30% of girls reported engaging in sex because a male was *too aroused* to stop, even if she didn't want to go forward.

Should we teach our daughters about hand jobs to protect them from poorly negotiated peer-pressure sex...or should we be able to help them feel empowered to say no? While the latter is more correct from our adult viewpoint, the former may be more natural for actual implementation in the teen world. And, of course, a "both/and" approach is probably most realistic.

One area for specific focus in negotiation skills is for girls who are on hormonal contraceptives, such as the pill. Young men may perceive this as "taking care of things" and therefore not want to wear a condom. These girls need help developing specific language to tell young men to use a condom. "I have a strict rule," the girl can say, "You must always wear a condom." In addition, we can teach our girls to remain strong (even if they are on the pill) by explaining to them that hormonal contraceptives change the function of the white blood cells in the woman's body and that recent studies have found that women on hormonal contraceptives have a much higher susceptibility at a cellular level to contracting STIs including HIV.

Radical Center Ruminations - If I had a daughter, I would be conflicted about supporting her use of hormonal contraceptives because of the changes they provoke in girls' bodies. Specifically, these medications have a strong negative impact on libido and sexual function, including increased vaginal dryness and pain during intercourse (sometimes leading to lifetime issues); an increased risk of chronic urinary tract infections; and an increased risk of contracting an STI. We will also discuss later the impact the pill can have on a woman's mate choice.

That said, if your daughter is on hormonal contraceptives for birth control or any other reason, make sure to role-play and model with her a situation in which a boy wants to have sex without a condom. Teach her to negotiate so that he still uses a condom. Help her to understand that it is in her best health interest to require this.

Social negotiations skills can be life saving for young gay men. The prevalence of unprotected anal intercourse among gay men who are diagnosed with HIV is still fairly high, at around 20-30%. Some of these men are having unprotected sex with other HIV positive men, but 16% are having unprotected sex with men of unknown HIV status and 13% with men of <u>known</u> HIV negative status (thus wittingly promoting exposure). Younger men may have less ability to say no to unprotected sex or may not be aware that the risk of HIV has not "gone away." You may need to clarify to these boys that they need to make a simple statement requesting condom use such as, "I'm sorry, I *always* use a condom."

Make sure all teenage boys (gay or straight or in-between) have a condom in their wallets and a backup box in their room. Storing condoms in the car isn't a good idea during the summer because the heat can weaken them. Although an unopened box of condoms has always been a great thing to see in our boys' closets, I have never wanted their lack of access to something as simple as this to be what allowed a life-changing pregnancy or disease into our family. Our strategy as parents has been to be open about sex, including protection, but to also make it very difficult for our teens to find a place to have sex. Being home alone and large SUV automobiles were not in our kids' stars.

Home Alone Equals Sexual Activity

As we parented through over a decade of teenaged boys in our home, I felt fortunate that our workplace had moved to a facility on our ranch so that either my husband or I was around almost all the time, providing supervision for our young men. Even when we knew we had sexually exploring teens, our goal was to make it difficult for them to find a place to regularly "go all the way" because research in sexual science is very clear about the role of supervision. Well-supervised adolescents have less high-risk, early and dangerous sex. Having a parent (and/or other adult) home after school reduces teen sexual behavior, lifetime sexual partner numbers and STI prevalence. Overall, young adults in families with more adult supervision significantly delay their sexual debut (loss of virginity). In one study of urban teens that spent most weekdays after school unsupervised each week, 42% of the boys had sex before age 14 and 9% of girls became active at this very young age. Most sexually active teens report having recently had sex in a home, 37% in their own and 43% in their partner's home. The more hours each week boys are unsupervised, the more sexual partners they end up having in high school. This effect is *three times stronger for boys* than girls, with 80% of boys who were unsupervised for over 30 hours a week being sexually active with multiple partners. Most fascinating, perhaps, in all these studies is what doesn't impact teen sexual activity. The following factors have no impact on teen sexual activity or their chances of developing STIs:

- Family structure (two parent versus one parent)

- Their school (public versus parochial/religious)

- Virginity pledges

- Assurances that they are not having sex

- Parents' attitudes towards adolescent sex (disapproving versus permissive).

The major factor that helps keep teens sexually healthy is whether an adult is physically present in the home. That is a fact that is worth addressing with action whether it means changing jobs, creating a community teen co-op (like many of us had with preschoolers) or hiring a "manny" to help with after school homework and activities.

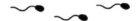

When it comes to teens and sex, human nature and human biology rule the day. Adolescents are biologic beings living out their internal nature. They are built for independence, high-risk experimentation and also the need for adult supervision. My assumption regarding my kids' sexual baseline was "they will have sex if we leave them unmonitored." Had I not spent my life studying human biology, I might have thought otherwise, but the truth is we cannot assume our teens are not having sex or that they are telling the truth about their sexual activities. However, we can help them make safer, more life affirming choices by being present in their lives and by not being afraid to speak truthfully to them. Vice Principal Todd Bender, at our local Ferris High School, best expressed guiding teens through decision making about sex when he said, "I don't tell kids they should or should not have sex. What I do tell them is that there will be people they trust to share their inner heart with, and that they shouldn't share 'down there' with anyone who they wouldn't also share 'up here' with, meaning their heart hopes and dreams." Ultimately, teaching sexual literacy and providing good supervision is about sharing with our kids our love for them and our own enjoyment of sex as mature adults. We want them to know that we have a vision for them, that they too will have enduring adult relationships full of intimacy and sexual satisfaction.

Chapter 3

Stalking The O

Soon after high school graduation I began moving toward my own adulthood, beginning with a cross-country trip to Tennessee with my friend Anna. Together, she and I set out from the Greyhound station in Seattle. With my "dirty red bandana" tied to my new red backpack I felt like Bobby McGee incarnate. Anna and I shared laughs and met some interesting people (mostly guys) as we traveled toward Nashville where I would start college at Vanderbilt University. Near Greeley, Colorado we decided to ditch the Greyhound and hitchhike up to Rocky Mountain Park. We planned to only catch rides with women or no more than one guy in a rig. This rule lasted about two hours in the hot summer sun. Five guys heading to the park in a white van welcomed us—and (luckily) later dropped us near a campground deep inside the park at dusk. The campground was full, so from there we hiked into the woods with no dinner and no tent—just our sleeping bags, a small blue tarp and a four-inch hunting knife. We were exhausted, and it was just dawning on us that maybe we needed a different plan.

The next day we went to the horse barn in the park that took tourists out on trail rides. Because we were both experienced horsewomen, we figured we would easily get jobs at the ranch. Unfortunately, the barn manager wasn't hiring, but we met some cute cowboys who worked there and we ended up staying with them for a week. One of them was Arnie, a dark Texan with a moustache and a drawl.

Every inch a working cowboy, he was also kind and gentle, as so many "tough" men actually are. I ended up snuggling with him in his bed in his cabin. Both he and I weren't interested in having intercourse (he not with a young virgin, me not *as* a young virgin), but he taught me about his body and my own in an unrushed, open way in the light of day and not hidden or cramped in a car like it had been in high school.

In retrospect, I see that he was trying to take me somewhere that I couldn't quite go—at least not yet. Because he was a gentleman, he put a lot of effort into my pleasure (even though I never orgasmed), and he also didn't mind that I had no idea what I was doing with and for him. It was the perfect platform to just enjoy skin on skin, tongue on skin and laughter in bed without feeling judged or dirty. When I left Arnie, he gave me a photo book on cowboys inscribed, "Well, hell, Joe—From a Real Cowboy—Love, Arnie." He and I stayed in touch for a while, but our worlds diverged as he went on to marry his high school sweetheart and become a rancher, and I went off to college at the preppy Vanderbilt University. I wish more young women could have an Arnie in their life to help teach them about their sexual self in a gentle unhurried way.

College was fun and busy as I studied my pre-veterinary classes with a minor in anthropology and began to realize my academic ability for the first time. I felt lucky to receive the top grade in freshman chemistry. The next year when I outscored all the other students in Vanderbilt's biochemistry course, I created a bit of a stir. My professor was stunned when I went in to pick up the exam. Shocked, he said, "I didn't know you were a girl. First time that's ever happened." Spelling my name "Joe" had paid off perhaps; I can't be sure I would have gotten that same grade if I had spelled my name Jo. I remember, years later, a female advisor on my PhD committee telling me to NEVER put my first name (as a woman) on any professional documents. To this day, all my *curriculum vitae* (resumes), grant applications and publications say "JE Ellington."

In the summer of my sophomore year in college, "it" finally happened. I met my first real lover on the Upper Peninsula of Michigan where I worked as a riding instructor at a summer camp. This was a dream job for me—getting up at 4:30 in the morning, feeding and tacking forty horses, riding all day, then heading to a local bar (a place very lax on their underage drinking policy) for hours of eating, drinking and laughing. I also met Duran, the head sailing instructor. Blonde, tan and a wonderful guitar player, Duran was four years older than me and was everything my vagabond self could want. Duran and I started hanging out. After several weeks, we decided it was time. Nervously, I set sail with him onto Lake Michigan, which is more like sailing on the ocean than a lake. Everything about the situation was neatly planned because we both had rigorous schedules with camper activities. In other words, we didn't have a lot of time.

As we skipped over the water, the sun shone on the lake's surface. Duran made a bed on the bottom of the boat and motioned me to come sit beside him, where things progressed naturally. Underneath me, the hardness of the wood floor hurt my spine and I felt an unpleasant stretching feeling internally. When we were done, I blurted out, "Well, that wasn't much fun." He laughed and said, "Just wait. It will be better next time." As we headed back, I felt disillusioned about the whole thing. But the next morning we decided to meet in my cabin during breakfast. Here we made love in the skinny lower bunk bed while everyone else was gone. This time it worked. I had my first orgasm! I knew nothing about orgasms, clitorises or arousal fluids, but as he began moving inside me, I felt a warm flooding sensation that made me gasp with wonder.

"What was that?" I asked.

He just laughed again and held me close.

Radical Center Ruminations - In cultures where female virginity is deemed necessary prior to marriage, a great deal of pressure is placed on the couple's wedding night. This often includes the need to show "first night" blood on the sheets as evidence of the bride's purity. Lest you think this custom has died out, in a recent 2007 survey of couples in their twenties presenting for sexual counseling in Turkey, 65% (two out of three!) were required to show the blood-stained sheet as proof of the woman's virginity their first night of marriage. But not all virgins bleed at their first intercourse. In fact, there is little published data to provide information as to the percentage of women who do so during this event. In a brief survey of medical professionals, only 34% of these women had a bloody "show" at their first intercourse—meaning that almost 2/3 of women did not.

When it comes to young women with intact hymens at first intercourse, only about 60% have this physical structure, meaning that almost half of all virgins don't have the intact hymen that men and their families seek as proof of purity. The outcome of failing to show evidence of virginal blood and an intact hymen after the first night can ruin lives and even lead to murder of the bride or members of her family. If the groom's family feels they have been cheated with an unchaste bride, they may take things into their own hands to cleanse their family honor.

Surgical hymen repair, especially with methods to promote bleeding after intercourse, is increasing in popularity. This is in large part due to the fact that it saves women's lives. Such hymen repair is credited in large part with an 80% decrease in "cleansing" murders over 10 years in Egypt.

Surgical repair of the hymen is debated (from different viewpoints) with regard to its ethical impact. In many countries it is illegal. A physician in Western countries where it is legal as a plastic surgery may wonder if it is "right" to do as it perpetuates gender social injustices. Sadly, over half of nonvirgin European women seeking hymen repair report a forced intercourse event in their lives leading to their need for the surgery. Hopefully, over time and with education, the test of virginal bleeding as proof of purity will go away. In large part, this change will need to be brought about by enlightened men in societies where it still matters.

Duran was patient and sensual, and I will be forever grateful that I was introduced to lovemaking by such a giving soul and an experienced lover even though our relationship didn't survive beyond the insular "summer loving" of camp life. Between him and my cowboy the year before, I had met two very fine men who taught me a sexual baseline of expecting both respectful treatment and effort toward my pleasure from grown men.

Losing my virginity that summer started me on a short-lived phase of sexual experimentation as I sought to learn who I was sexually and what worked to turn me on. Now that I knew what an orgasm felt like, I found several ways to find one, alone or with someone else. In fact, I realized orgasms were one of my favorite parts of being human!

The Big O in Women – Who Cares?

The idea of writing this book to help people decipher the available information on sexual science came to me a few years ago as I lay in a hotel room in Palm Springs, sick with the flu during a winter vacation. Through the wall, I heard a couple having sex that only lasted about two minutes. "How frustrating!" I thought, as I pictured the woman who obviously didn't orgasm (from what I heard). I wondered what the couple had done to help deal with the man's premature ejaculation and also pondered (as I have many times before) the question thousands of scientists have asked: "Why do women orgasm?" It is obvious that men must orgasm in order for children to be conceived, but there isn't much evidence that females in other species have orgasms, with the exception of approximately eight primate species. Many scientists and lay people alike have often wondered why human women are one of these lucky few.

Because female orgasm is not required for reproduction, its sole purpose appears to be ensuring that sex is enjoyable for women. This is a fascinating aspect of human biology, one that we don't explore often enough. Understanding that an *entire organ evolved in humans solely for sexual pleasure of the woman* stands in marked contrast to the misogynistic teachings around sexuality of the past 10,000 years. So let's explore the female orgasm a bit, looking at its role over the hundreds of thousands of years our species has been around.

Unlike humans, most ovulating female mammals are driven to have sex by high estrogen levels when they are "in heat." These females seek out sexual partners as a physical response to chemical and hormone shifts in their bodies even though they never have an orgasm to reward them for the act. In contrast, women accept and even seek intercourse with men at any time of the month and not just when they are ovulating. So, lying in my hotel bed with a fever, I thought, "There has to be an evolutionary reason for orgasms in women. Somehow the ability of the man to maintain an erection long enough to give a woman an orgasm must be a beneficial selection trait for men, making them more desired and sought after by women and allowing them to father more children." My mind started to wander to a time before "culture" and marriage in the 200,000 plus years *Homo sapiens* have been on earth. We girls must have looked for the men who could make us feel so good that we would keep going back for more sex until we conceived. Somehow a woman's orgasm had an evolutionary benefit for our species or our bodies wouldn't have developed this seemingly "unnecessary" organ. "Yes," I thought as I remembered that first orgasm with Duran, that orgasm made me want to keep having sex with him!

The Nitty Gritty on Orgasms

Orgasm in both sexes results in an oxytocin (bonding chemical) release, as muscles contract, and a dopamine (pleasure chemical) flood of the brain. In orgasm, we feel sensations throughout our body like few other human experiences. Research shows that over 80% of Western women have experienced an orgasm sometime in their lives, and 75% have had an orgasm at least once during intercourse. These studies also confirm that the quality of sex a woman experiences dramatically impacts her chances of orgasm. In fact, up to 70% of the variation in women's frequency of orgasm during sex may be due to *external* environmental factors, including sexual skills and physical aspects of her partner, the science of which you will likely find fascinating. I know I did!

The percentage of women who regularly orgasm during "vaginal intercourse" (i.e., penile-vaginal intercourse) ranges from about 40% for younger gals to less than 30% for older women. For men, the situation is *profoundly* different, with 90% of younger and 75% of older men routinely reaching orgasm during partnered sex. This makes sense since no male orgasm equals no conception. Thus, orgasm *is* the natural climax to sex for men.

Perhaps not surprisingly, although most women don't routinely orgasm during penile-vaginal intercourse, up to *80% of women who have partnered sex with other women do regularly orgasm.* To a great extent, this is likely related to an understanding among women as to how to touch and stimulate the female clitoris (not too soft, not too hard, "just right"). Indeed, a woman's inability to orgasm in partnered sex is often due to "operator error." Women who have to masturbate after intercourse to find release already know this. These findings tell us that a woman's ability to orgasm is highly correlated to her partner choice, not an intrinsic capability inside her. *All women with normal clitoral anatomy and physiology have the ability to orgasm.* Not all (and in fact not most) penile-vaginal intercourse between men and women leads to a female orgasm. To better understand why something all women have (a clitoris) only "works" (resulting in orgasm) sometimes, let's start by reviewing the anatomy and physiology of the organ.

The Anatomy of the Clitoris

In our society, few of us are taught the true makeup of this female orgasm organ. Perhaps the most prevalent myth in human society about the clitoris is with regard to its location and size, specifically that most of us think that the external glans (the "nub," or "head") IS the clitoris. In actuality, this is just the tip of a much larger iceberg of an organ that lies under and around our entire vulva and urethra. Anatomically, *most* of the clitoris lies deep beneath the fat and muscle of the vulva where it is attached to the front of our pubic area and on both sides of the vulvar lips. Pretty much any place we put pressure on in this area can feel good. Evolutionary biology suggests that somewhere in the last 300,000 years, natural selection

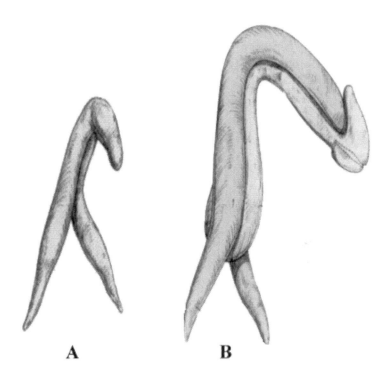

A   **B**

The erectile tissue of the: A) clitoris, showing the external "nub" or glans (as the tip of the hook), the larger body and the roots that split along each side of the vulva; and B) penis. Anatomic similarities are unmistakable. (Reproduced with permission from Puppo 2011 and 2014.)

experimented with developing this large organ underneath our female skin as primates moved from mammalian sex during "heat" to being sexually receptive all month long. For reasons mainly of pleasure assurance, the clitoris developed with a boomerang shape that measures about *five* inches long from front to back along both sides of the genital opening; deep to the skin about *two to three* inches; and lying at least that wide from side to side across both sides of the vulva. The woman's clitoris is essentially the same size as a man's penis, but with 90% of the arousal tissue being *under* the skin surrounding the vulva.

This clitoris is made out of erectile cells that enlarge when aroused (like the penis...again, the penis is actually a male external version of the female's internal clitoris). It also developed sensitivity to estrogen and testosterone sex steroids in order to help maintain function. We know that the clitoris came into being, in some part, to make sure people had sex for conception because in women who go through menopause (and are done reproducing) the clitoral cells begin to die. When these same women take hormone replacement therapy (which tricks our bodies into thinking we are still reproductively active) this atrophy or cell death of the clitoral arousal tissue is stopped.

Overall, female sexual response involves the clitoris and the distal (outer most) urethra and vagina, all three forming a unified "cluster" that becomes engorged with blood during sexual arousal. The infamous G spot (or other unique pleasure places in the literature) when studied by MRI is not a separate part of female anatomy from the clitoris—it is part of the cluster of organs that respond with increased blood flow during sexual stimulation (the "arousal tissue").

One would think that this anatomy would be well taught, but in reality the clitoris keeps getting lost, even in medical textbooks. In contrast to the many pages devoted to penile anatomy, detailed information for the clitoris has been lacking, even in classics like *Gray's Anatomy* (which many doctors use in their training). Thankfully, the feminists of the '70s forced textbooks to be corrected, and somewhat more accurate information has been added to the literature. Nevertheless, even today, modern textbooks often misplace aspects of this organ, making it difficult for healthcare providers to understand its true physiology and size.

Radical Center Ruminations - The female clitoris evolved to provide women pleasure so they would want to have sex and would conceive. If female sexual fulfillment is feared, one way

to deal with an organ that has no use other than pleasure is to remove it. Approximately 140 million women alive today have undergone female genital mutilation (FGM) to narrow the vagina and remove portions of the clitoris and/or vulva. This is equivalent to 45% of the U.S. population. I wanted to bring this topic up because only about half of women who have undergone this procedure know that surgical reconstruction may be a pathway to a better sex life for them. Every year an estimated 3 million girls go through the procedure, and in some countries up to 20% of girls die from complications. In many countries it is viewed as equivalent to male circumcision and thus is called "female circumcision" as a part of the ritual to maturity. Of course, removing the male foreskin can improve a man's sexual sensitivity, rather than destroy it as does this "female circumcision."
The age for the FGM procedure can be as young as five. The procedure varies in severity from Type III which cuts and seals the labia of the vulva to create a narrower opening, to Type II with removal of the clitoral glans and the inner labia, to Type I with full excision of the deep clitoral structures surrounding the vulva and the outer vulvar labia. In contrast to Western medicine's ignorance of true clitoral anatomy, the people who perform Type I genital mutilation fully understand the depth and breadth of a woman's clitoral arousal tissues.

A recent study reviewed success among genital mutilation survivors in France who went through reconstructive surgery. Shockingly, 20% of these women had undergone the FGM illegally in France. The report found that reconstructive surgery for women with Type II and Type III FGM was highly beneficial. Specifically,

35% of women who never had orgasms before surgery were able to afterwards. Half the women who had had restricted orgasm (small ones) had greater intensity orgasms afterward, although a minority (20%) of women had worse orgasm potential after surgery. The good news is that sexual fulfillment improved for over 80% of women, and 30% had a reduction in pain at sex.

Surgery can only repair a potential. Women who have undergone the most radical Type I procedures may have limited tissues to repair. Couples that include a woman who has had FGM and are interested in improving their sexual intimacy should discuss the reconstructive procedure with their physician. Many husbands may not be as adverse to their wives enjoying sexuality as is culturally assumed. The group Equality Now is working to improve laws and the justice system to bring about an end to this practice of removing something that human evolution spent years building into women for our greater good and joy.

Perhaps one of the reasons (along with sexism) that the clitoris hasn't received appropriate attention is that scientists have not been sure how it, and the orgasms it gives women, benefitted human sexual biology. They were and still are asking the same question I asked in the hotel room. Given the fact that many women do not experience vaginal orgasms, it makes sense that both scientists and lovers have had difficulty understanding this organ. In trying to figure out the role of the clitoris, some scientists and sexual therapists have debated (with hundreds of published articles on countless hours of research) the pros and cons of different types of female orgasm. However, many scientists like me have come to realize that these discussions are somewhat ridiculous. The fact is that all female orgasms following *any* contact of the genital area are orgasms triggered by and through the clitoral complex arousal tissues. It is not possible to penetrate, touch or lick this pubic region of women without contacting the clitoris. Discussions of what feels best and is most fulfilling for individual women is a matter of preference regarding the type of stimulation that most easily triggers her to climax. In actuality, there is no anatomical evidence for a "vaginal orgasm" separated from the clitoris because it isn't physically possible. All orgasms arise from clitoral response.

What Good Are Unreliable Orgasms?

Sexual science shows us that female orgasm is very important to how both men and women feel about their relationship quality. During partnered sex, higher frequency and intensity of female orgasm explains at least 10% of the variability in *overall female relationship satisfaction*. And in women for whom sexual satisfaction is a high priority (count me in), the percentage impact of female orgasm on the marriage quality is even higher. For men, the female partner's orgasm frequency and intensity also relate to how he feels about the couple's sexual compatibility and thus his overall relationship satisfaction. Contrary to what we sometimes think, our guys like living with us better when they can please us, make us happy and keep us engaged and interested in sex.

If everyone feels better when we gals orgasm, why is this event so damn elusive for some of us? What we are learning now is that having the clitoris and female orgasm evolve to be finicky and a bit unreliable was of evolutionary benefit for our species as a whole. Female orgasm became a method of mate selection for women, to help them choose the *right* man so that their offspring would be the strongest and most healthy children possible.

Female Orgasm Helped Women Choose the Best Dad

It makes evolutionary sense that female orgasm plays a larger role than just to provide great sex for us girls individually. For the clitoris to have come into existence, it had to provide an overall benefit for our species as a whole. It appears that whether or not a woman had an orgasm with a man instinctually helped our great-great-great-...grandmothers choose the best fathers for their babies. New understanding from several fields of science suggests that as female orgasm became possible through an expanding clitoral organ, males who were genetically superior could more consistently trigger the orgasm in women. This made sex with these men more fun, leading the ladies to seek them out for the repeated intercourse required for conception. A female's orgasmic response to a man was related to his outward characteristics (his *phenotype*) which reflected his internal genetic quality (his *genotype*).

In short, the men who were "hot" to our great-great-great-... grandmothers also had the best quality genes ("high value genes"). Better genes evolutionarily are those that carry the strongest immune systems and have the least variation and mutation (e.g., damaged portions of genes). Having these super strong genes from the dad passed on to a woman's offspring best ensured her babies' survival. A man's ability to bring a woman to orgasm during intercourse served the same purpose as does the peacock's tail in attracting the peahen. Both are instinctual cues of the male's genetic quality. And just like the females of any species, women subconsciously sought, and still seek, these high-genetic-value mates to father their children for the best chance of healthy offspring.

Over the eons, each species has developed its own unique *mating strategy* for choosing these best partners for mating and reproduction. Mating strategies are what allow a species to evolve because through their influence, females choose males to reproduce with that result in robust babies who survive to become adults and parents themselves. While we get a kick out of some of the mating strategies out there, such as bugs and birds that look odd or do fancy dances, growing evidence suggests that female orgasm developed as a similar selection tool for women to choose (biologically) who should father their children.

Even today, we find that humans haven't outgrown this ancient biological mating strategy. The attractiveness of a present-day man as rated by third-party scientists can predict *a woman's probability of orgasm* with this man. And women who partner with higher masculinity men (the *"dominant male"*) report more frequent and easier orgasms during vaginal intercourse than do women with less masculine men. This is because a man's attractiveness (his facial symmetry and muscle patterns) are not only skin deep. They also reflect his gene quality and ability to provide his offspring with inherited immunity to diseases and a stronger chance for survival. Nature provided women a functional (and fun), subconscious way to ensure the dads with the best genes fathered the most kids.

Over the generations women chose the sexy looking guys who happened to be better able to give her an orgasm during intercourse, so she came back for more sex until she was pregnant and gave birth to strong babies who inherited dad's high quality genes. Masculine looks and sexual prowess are passed on from fathers to sons, making it easy to see how this type of man stamped his presence on our species over time and helped drive development of the clitoris and the somewhat quirky female orgasms.

In contrast, if women had reached orgasm every time they had vaginal intercourse (with only a 20% chance of becoming pregnant each month), nothing would have pushed moms to find the best Baby Daddy for the follow-up sexual encounters required for conception. The orgasm developed as an instinctual mate selection tool to give us babies that could survive the tough natural world in which we humans lived. And as women's bodies evolved to develop the clitoris and the capacity to orgasm, men's bodies also evolved to better give us this pleasure.

Size and Duration Matter for Female Orgasm

Men with stronger genes, as manifest in a classically male masculine body type and facial characteristics, are not only hot. They also have better "equipment" for leading women to orgasm. Their good genes correlate with a larger penis, higher testosterone levels and longer lasting erections. A woman's ability to orgasm during penile-vaginal intercourse is, at least in part, a factor of her partner's phenotype (physical characteristics). Although we are often told that penile size doesn't matter, surveys of women around the world have found it does, during penile-vaginal intercourse. A *majority* of women prefer penises that are larger. For instance, in an Internet survey of 26,000 heterosexual women, 94% of women who had a partner with a large penis reported they were very sexually satisfied. Only 32% of women whose partners had small penises reported being very sexually satisfied. In these studies, size mattered, but it mattered more to women who frequently orgasm during penile-vaginal intercourse (PVI) than for women who orgasm during other kinds of sex play (e.g., cunnilingus). This suggests a relationship between a man with a large penis and the ability of his female partner to easily orgasm during PVI. This makes sense if we recall the anatomy of the clitoris. A larger penis can contact more of the erectile tissue complex, giving more pleasure stimulation. In contrast, frequency of orgasms during other types of sex (non-PVI) didn't differ between women who thought size mattered and those who didn't. Women can orgasm from many types of sexual contact, giving other routes to pleasure for them with partners who are less well endowed. But for our ancestresses, men with larger penises were part of the whole package (so to speak) that brought them back for more reproductive sex.

Penile size and testosterone levels in the male are highly heritable. Once again, dads who made the ladies happy would have had *more* sex resulting in *more* pregnancies and the fathering of *more* sons. These sons would have also carried on traits of high testosterone and sexual prowess through subsequent generations as *more* of their high-gene-quality boys lived to adulthood and fatherhood. In the end, a positive evolutionary selection benefit for our species became linked to these masculine, sexually successful men (i.e., they equaled more, more, more).

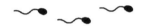

Not only penile size but also the length of time a man can keep an erection impacts female orgasm. Similar to the man on the other side of the wall in my Palm Springs hotel room, up to 20% of men at any age have premature ejaculation (PE), with ejaculation occurring within two minutes of vaginal penetration. In fact, we can learn a good deal of fascinating science from this medical condition. For example, a link has been found between stronger quality genes for immunity to diseases and how long a man can maintain an erection. Specifically, men with PE have more genetic variation and more genes associated with lower immunity status than men with longer erection times.

This finding further supports a functional role of female orgasm. Here is how. Studies show that there is an association between how long a man can maintain his erection and the likelihood that a woman will orgasm during penile-vaginal intercourse. Only about 25% of women climax with vaginal intercourse of two minutes or less while 60% of women orgasm with intercourse lasting over ten minutes. For comparison, the average time it takes women to orgasm when they masturbate is four minutes. Men who can't provide an erection for at least four minutes are highly disadvantaged in helping their partner reach orgasm during vaginal intercourse. If our ancestresses chose to have repeated intercourse less frequently with men who had a shorter time to ejaculation (and carried the related lower quality immune system genes), they would have also conceived fewer children with these men. This would have lessened the presence of genes for low immunity in the population overall, which would have been a benefit for the society as a whole. Although these immunity genes may not matter as much now, they could have made the difference between survival and death in our distant past.

Female Orgasms Are Perfect Just The Way They Are!

Looking at it this way, the hit or miss nature of orgasms in women causes individuals a great deal of stress, but in actuality their demanding nature is perfect for the health of our species. In order for women to orgasm during reproductive sex, our evolved mating strategies required the following parameters be met for babies to be made:

- Both partners had to be in good health.

- The environment had to be conducive to sex, without "fight or flight" stress.

- The couple needed to respond to each other's physical and social cues.

- The man needed to be a genetic stud to please momma or she would look elsewhere.

A quick review of this list shows that all these factors optimize the future success of any children born to this pair as well! The female orgasm was the *perfect* selection criteria for humans when deciding if we were in the right place and social structure to have a new baby.

Although the last few thousand years have continuously asserted the patriarchal notion that women do not, or should not, enjoy sex, our natural and biological sciences show just the opposite. Because human females are sexually receptive all month long and not just during their fertile time, women could (and still do) "audition" men in trial sex. If the man pleased her *consciously* with an orgasm, as an *unconscious* indicator of his better gene strength, she would then have continued having sex with him until she ovulated and conceived.

It is important to remember that although nature likes the masculine and muscular dominant male because he consistently fathers the strongest offspring with regard to survival, gene variations are also valuable to a species. These are what have allowed us to adapt and become who we are today. Not all genetic variability is bad. Bill Gates may not have been "King of the Hill" back in the day, but his genes are allowing me to word process this book! There is room for all kinds of men and lovers in life, but understanding why we are attracted to different people can be empowering for both men and women.

Even today it is important to understand how our human mating strategies can still impact us. Women continue to seek out these highly *masculine* males, sometimes out of the blue, when they are fertile (ovulating) or for extramarital affairs. This is because we are wired to look for male partners (via eons of human history) in which "good genes" are the more masculine ones. We naturally are attracted to these good-gene males, at least at certain points of our lives (e.g., when we are young or when we are most fertile), in part through the gift of orgasm from sex with these men.

The Dominant Male in Fiction and Fantasy

Although not all ladies experiencing a mid-life crisis will run off with James Bond, many of us are nonetheless drawn to the dominant male in fiction and fantasy. Recent studies show that female sexual fantasies incorporating a dominant man increase a woman's sexual arousal and orgasm rates. This is because our fictional "bad boy" is the archetypal masculine man that evolutionary biology leaves us wanting, as we seek his powerful genes. The more masculine the man, the more he instinctively attracts our mating brains. Again, remember, this genetic superiority in alpha masculinity predates our present morality and social systems and has been at work through 95% of our human history (excluding the past 10,000 years). In the past, survival of our genes as a species required more masculinity not less, hence our ongoing, unconscious attraction to these types of men.

Romance novels along these lines are "hard-wired reading" for many women. These novels always include a handsome, masculine and dangerous man...yummy! These "heroes" are the dominant male. Their plot is usually one of "Adversary Transformation" in which the conflict is between the heroine and her dominant sexual adversary. Eventually the heroine conquers this man's heart through her beauty and charm, seducing him into love and a commitment. She then transforms his character without diminishing his masculinity. Most types of women choose to read romance novels (including feminists) for the enjoyment, excitement and sexual arousal they provide.

Romance novels are a lot like female sexual fantasies, which are really just self-generated erotic stories. Interestingly, many romance books written by women for women include the rape or domination of the female lead. Many women also find fantasies of forced sex exciting and sexually arousing. A review of 20 studies into the role of rape fantasies in women's sexual lives consistently found that over 40% of women had rape fantasies. On average, about 14% of women use rape fantasies as their preferred sexual fantasy, and most women rate these scenarios in their top ten fantasies. The prevalence of rape fantasies for sexual arousal has remained consistent over the past four decades (since their first study), likely because these fantasies improve sexual self-fulfillment in women.

Married women who use frequent rape fantasies report more marital contentment and sexual fulfillment including orgasm. In contrast, women who reported no fantasies at all were more likely to have difficulty with sexual arousal and orgasm. And women who identify with feminist values are just as likely to have rape fantasies as other women. The use of rape fantasies by sexually healthy, satisfied women suggests that these "stories" inside our minds are just one more expression of normal sexuality.

Some of the current theories as to why women find rape fantasy sexually arousing include their ritualistic display of male dominance and female surrender, rooted in our biologic mating strategies. Specifically, women may have an evolutionary drive to select, engage and then submit to a high quality, dominant male. It needs to be clear here that human rape fantasies are not a desire for actual rape. Rape would decrease the woman's reproductive success by allowing unselected men to father her children. But if she selects a strong, dominant man, as proven by a subconscious pursuit and conquering ritual, such "submission" would be advantageous for her offspring.

Many women in consensual, happy relationships engage in private rape fantasies. For almost half of all women, this fantasy scenario serves to increase sexual arousal and increase attraction to their real life partners. It is normal, and it isn't anything you need to share with anyone else!

The Faked Female Orgasm

In contrast to real orgasms which make couples happier, faked female orgasm is associated with less male and female sexual and relationship satisfaction. In other words, both women and men like it when women have real orgasms. Men with women who fake can tell this accurately about a third of the time, and it tends to make the man less sexually satisfied in their relationship. In this regard, faked female orgasm serves neither the man nor the woman.

Have you ever faked an orgasm? I have, and I'm not alone. In a recent study of orgasm habits, 58% of women reported faking an orgasm at least some of the time; meanwhile, men reported faking orgasms during sex 21% of the time (yes, guys fake it too). The researchers also found that women who fake orgasms are *more* likely to be sexually unfaithful to their husband or boyfriend, perhaps because of a lack of sexual satisfaction? Faking orgasms also has another negative effect on women—the likelihood that these women will have a real orgasm with a partner significantly declines. It is hard to tell him what to do right if he doesn't even know he is doing something wrong!

If you are mostly faking orgasms during love making, know that there are many resources to help you move beyond this, many of which I discuss in this book. The scariest part is telling your partner and explaining that you want to learn together how to find more fulfilling sex for you. A gentle way to do this is to tell him that you have "started" faking it more because you don't want to pressure him but that you would prefer to find new ways to improve your sexual responsiveness. Let the past go, but start experimenting, reading and finding videos. And reinvent your solo time in masturbation. The more you orgasm, the higher your testosterone will be and the more sexually responsive you will feel.

To help you move from faking to real orgasms, there are two schools of thought. I suggest that you read and learn about both to see which works best for you. The first is the "no vibrator" camp, and no one teaches this better than the venerable Betty Dodson (*dodsonandross. com*). Thousands of women sing Betty's praises. The other is Team Vibrator. At Adam & Eve's website take their Vibrator Wizard survey to find the best vibrator for you. Whichever you choose, order the book, the video or the vibrator. You don't need to keep faking it!

The Inner Truth

Although women in hot pursuit of a dominant male aren't registering the biology of our mating strategies, it may be helpful at times to point out this "behind the scenes" instinctual attraction. By understanding that our DNA wants this man's good genes in order to optimize the health of our potential offspring, we can also realize that this guy might not actually be the best man for us long term. Talking frankly about evolutionary biology and mating strategies can be immensely helpful because they are, from the scientific viewpoint, our "inner truth." While we don't operate only in response to these instincts (other biological and social cues hold sway), they are part of our inherent humanness. Explaining "bad boy" instincts to young women (or women in transition) can help them at least understand their wiring. It can empower women to realize that they actually do control who they mate with and need sensual self awareness to direct their own sexual paths. This journey can include training *different* types of men in what we need as women so that we don't over-rely on a particular definition of a man for our sexual and romantic fulfillment.

Chapter 4

The Lovers We Choose

Of course, I knew nothing about human mating strategies and how women instinctually select the right man when I was in my twenties. I wish I had. Although it may not have changed the course of my life, I would have at least perhaps paused to measure the steps I took during this decade against the backdrop of our evolved human nature.

After getting a bit wild my first two years at Vanderbilt, the pendulum of my identity then swung back to my roots as I realized it was time to start dating men who shared my spiritual values. One fall weekend, I went on a retreat to the Smokey Mountains with a group of young people from my church. A friend's brother, Jay, who had recently graduated from Harvard, came along. Jay was a tall, blonde Irishman, with classical masculine features (he would later go on to become a model). He was also a talented musician and singer. Sitting around the campfire, our singing voices blended together so well we immediately thought of ourselves as a duo. Over the next several months, we fell in love through long-distance letters and quick weekend visits to each other's homes. Because of our faith commitment, physical activity was limited to kissing and snuggling.

This was an exciting time in my life. I still recall getting the white letter of acceptance from the University of Tennessee Veterinary School. I had applied for early admission after just three years of undergraduate studies. When the letter came, I held the envelope for a good ten minutes before opening it. Finally I ripped it open and started screaming—"I'm in, I'm in!" After telling my parents, I called Jay and we celebrated over the phone. Later that year, on my 21st birthday, Jay proposed to me. As was the norm during that time in our lives, we felt a higher calling guiding our decision—yet, more than we realized, we were also following our hormones and youthful mating instincts.

Eight months later, a week before our wedding in August, Jay drove out to meet me in Washington State for our big day. When he arrived, I took him aside and told him I was having serious second thoughts. With family and friends coming in from around the country and even from overseas, we talked and prayed, and finally convinced ourselves again that it was the right plan. Some deep inner truths were surfacing for me, but I chose not to listen. While I loved and respected Jay, I also felt boxed in by our faith, our sense of duty and, honestly, by the three hundred guests who were coming to unite us.

We did go through with the wedding, and like first weddings often are, ours was an amazing celebration. The church, filled to capacity with our guests, uplifted us all. At the flower-surrounded altar, with my father presiding, Jay sang a song he had written for me.

"Joanna my chosen, Joanna my bride."

There were few dry eyes in the church. However, all this joy aside, soon after our service, my father commented that during the ceremony there was a lot about God and very little about our being in love with each other. His words would come back to me several times over the next seven years.

My father (as an experienced marriage counselor and pastor) gave Jay and I his frank, practical advice on sex within marriage, words

I still remember: "It doesn't matter if you orgasm at the same time or not; this is overrated." Both Jay and I had some experience in intimacy, but none as husband and wife, so we welcomed advice from more experienced mentors. But nothing could have prepared us for the sexual mishaps that, sadly, began from our first day of marriage. Perhaps instead of all the china we received, we would have been better off with a copy of *The Joy of Sex*!

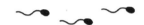

During the first night and the next several days of our honeymoon on the Oregon Coast, we made love several times a day. I am physically very small (everywhere). Also, I had started on oral contraceptives, not knowing they would profoundly change my sexual physiology for the worse. On our wedding night, I was exhausted from coordinating the huge ceremony and reception. There wasn't much natural lubrication to be had. The sex started out uncomfortable and went to extremely painful as we kept "practicing" to try to get it right. By the third day, I was in such constant burning pain that I would start crying when we made love.

But we both wanted me to orgasm. We decided we just needed to keep working at it. The more we tried, the more I couldn't find release, and the more sore I became. In tears, I called my best friend from high school who had more sexual experience than me. Logically, she suggested we use a lubricant. Back in those days, there was one—the tube of K-Y® Jelly that hid in everyone's bedside table drawer. That day, we went to the store and bought some. Excited, we rushed back to our cabin to try sex while using it. But the lubricant made me *more* inflamed, not less. I did not know then that K-Y Jelly (like most lubricants) has a salt (ion) concentration approximately six times that of our bodily fluids, so it can be like putting salt water in your eyes if you are irritated or sensitive to its formula. My vulva and clitoris became even more red and raw after applying the lubricant.

Assuming something was wrong with me as a woman, I started to feel a certain amount of sexual dysfunction. I was sexually frustrated too and became aggressive and short with Jay. It never occurred to me to masturbate to relieve the sexual tension that was growing in my body. These difficult experiences with sex would later become an inspiration for the scientific work I ended up dedicating my life to. In a sense, I am glad they happened, but at the time, they were completely demoralizing.

Finally, I did have an orgasm after several weeks, and we both cheered with relief! Although I thought, at the time, that my choice of Jay as a mate took place with my rationale mind and my romantically inclined heart, in truth he fit the ticket for every girl's instinctual dream date. He was a physically attractive, masculine man, as well as charming and respectful. He embodied what my hormones and instincts wanted, so I selected him, not understanding that our mating strategies, as ancient and cellular as women themselves, don't always mesh with our marriage goals.

The Hidden World of Mating Strategies and Sexual Selection

Mating has existed among our ancestors for a million years or more, but the thoughts and feelings we call love and marriage are a modern phenomenon, emerging over the past ten thousand years. Again mating strategies are the instinctual brain's attraction and sex drive that dictate how the *individual* chooses a partner in reproduction. No matter who you are, your cells remember how to mate even though they may not be sure what love is or what marriage looks like. Whereas the ability to successfully love and be loved can take decades to learn, the subconscious map for mating is inside all of us, all the time. In my case, instinctually, I had a young woman's inner map for how to select a man, and Jay had all the characteristics of a dominant male in this regard, one who would likely father highly capable offspring. My choice of a partner to mate with was also driven by many millennia of human *sexual selection*. This selection process over time has defined which types of men are the best for fathering the strongest offspring within our environment and human social structures. Women like masculine, strong men, but we could have just as easily have evolved to prefer men who sang a certain kind of song, or had a thick shaggy ruff of hair down their back, or built a specific type of house for us.

Sexual selection is the evolutionary mechanism by which a species chooses who will be the parents that bring forward the next generation, in contrast to the mating strategy as it selects the individual person our DNA is drawn to. Specifically, sexual selection determines what is "hot or not" for that species. By being one of the species that evolved for our males to be larger and stronger than our females, we know that men had to compete vigorously with each other to gain access to fertile women.

Why Are Men Bigger Than Women?

For most species where males and females work intimately together in single pairs to raise the young, the two sexes do not differ much in how they look or in their size (think of Emperor penguins). In contrast, in species where groups of females are fertile at the same time and males compete for the right to breed these female "harems," the sexual selection process over time leads to sexual dimorphism, meaning differences in appearance, strength and size of males and females, such as that seen in primates, including humans.

The development of: 1) strong, muscular and combative men and 2) a reproductive cycle that triggers groups of women to be fertile and have their periods at the same time (which any father of girls can attest to) both reflect the competitive sexual selection process that humans evolved with and through.

Our ancestors' dominant males were constantly competing for the sexually receptive females, and new younger-better-faster-stronger males consistently challenged the existing dominant male for this right. In fact, if you were to "create" your own most successful species for a sci-fi novel, you would most likely create this kind of situation. Sexual selection ensures that the *best, highest quality genes* in a given time and environment are always getting moved forward into the next generation, helping species adapt to a changing world.

On a continuum of how sexual selection impacts the social interactions between males, humans are luckier than many other species for whom options come down to a choice between reproducing or dying. For example, among elephant seals, only *one male will father 90% of the seal pups* in a given area. The battles between these males for the female harems are bloody and often fatal. Human beings are not elephant seals nor are we the more cooperative Emperor penguins. We fall somewhere in between. And like for many other males, dominance among men doesn't always require a physical battle. Just as the lion can subconsciously register the size of another lion's mane (an outward sign of his testosterone level and dominance) or the deer may check out his rivals' antlers, men (like other animal males) can make a decision to stand and fight or to walk away unharmed. Men constantly use subconscious rituals and physical cues, such as assessing the muscle definition and size of the man who just whistled at his girlfriend, to determine whether it is in their best interest to battle for dominance or to submit. By choosing not to fight every challenge (i.e., not being like the elephant sea lions), survival rates for men improved over time, allowing more of them to be around to function in support of the human social structure.

Over time, competition between males through strength, became an inherent aspect of being a man, just as the male elephant grows tusks or a bower bird makes an elaborate nest. A lot of what we see around us with regards to human "male" behavior and competition actually links back to sexuality. Men have to compete to be selected by women as sexual partners, and remember we gals will be instinctually drawn to that dominant male, the strongest most competitive man.

Women are the "Deciders"

A key factor for species that have intense competition between males for the right to procreate is that the females *control* day-to-day access to sex. As women, we are historically far more empowered than we often have been led to believe. I am speaking here of our power throughout human history and not just the past ten thousand years of recorded patriarchal history. It is important to remember that prehistoric *Homo sapiens* who lived over two hundred thousand years ago, had the same genes that we have today. They did not differ from us by the 1% that modern dogs and wolves do in their DNA. *Homo sapiens* were us and we are them! What we consider as human "history" (since the rise of agriculture and patriarchal culture) is actually less than 5% of our human time on earth.

Looking through the lens of evolutionary biology and anthropology, the sexual selection traits in humans and our mating strategies confirm that ancient women controlled the basis of human survival and development—they determined who they would have sex with. It makes sense that women needed to be as choosy as possible when it came to who would father their children. Pregnancy and child rearing "cost" a woman much more in time and body requirements (to carry a pregnancy and nurse a baby) than babymaking costs a man.

Though we all tend to think we make romantic choices out of "love above," we do not, especially when we are on a hormone high, such as during puberty and a woman's fertile time of the month. Our current stage of history is offering unique challenges to the ancient mating and sexual selection strategies that have brought us this far to-date. One of the largest of these challenges has also been a key factor in unlinking the biologic reality that sexuality equals reproduction. While oral contraceptives ("the pill") have brought us sexual freedom, equality for women and economic strength (through delayed childbirth), they have also had a significant impact on our instinctual mating and selection systems, sometimes for the worse.

Mate Selection and the Pill: The Cost of Fooling Mother Nature

I had no idea in 1981 that starting oral contraceptives (OC) would play a major role in ruining my first marriage. However, when I saw the difference in how my body functioned sexually before taking the pill, while taking it, and then again once off OC, I knew for me the pill was bad, bad news (this would later become a subject I wanted to study during my PhD training). At 21, I was a young "experiment of one" who, along with more than *80%* of American women, had used the pill at one point in her life. Over half of women who use the pill or other similar hormonal contraceptive do so in their mate selection years, between 16 to 34 years of age, just as I did. But I did not realize that OCs lead to increased health problems, such as chronic genital pain, depression and bipolar disease. They can also affect mate selection by interfering with our highly evolved mating strategies. Let's look at how this happens.

During the normal six days of the month when women are fertile and ovulation is near, gals unconsciously shift their mental imagery of the type of man they are attracted to. They are more drawn to the independent, hunky and dominant male with his high-value genes—they like his face, his body shape, his smell, his voice and even his chest thumping (episodes of displaying dominance among other men). Women prefer this type of man when they are fertile without realizing it, through smell and sight, including his cues of attractiveness and facial symmetry (all supporting his good genes).

Interestingly, fertile women also prefer a man whose face is visually *dissimilar* to their own face, meaning men who are unrelated to them and therefore, look different from the woman. During mate selection for sex that could lead to reproduction (such as when we are ovulating) women choose to be with high-genetic value men, who carry a gene set differing most dramatically from their own. Once again the external physical appearance (that phenotype) of the face is subconsciously telling women about the internal genetic characteristics of this man she is courting. A man who looks different in appearance from a woman will have a more divergent immune system from her (specifically, that of the Major Histocompatibility Complex or MHC) than a man who looks like her. This MHC is crucial for human health and function. Therefore, when we are fertile we instinctually choose men who will ensure the strongest immune system and best future survival for our babies.

After ovulation, once our estrogen levels decline, ladies quickly switch to preferring to be around men who are *coalitional*, meaning not as dominant. These are the men who enjoy functioning in a larger social group and are less competitive than the dominant male. Additionally, we prefer men who are genetically "more like us," with similar facial resemblance and similar immune MHC genes. By coding this cycle into our female DNA, nature seems to encourage us to seek out related male kin (noncompetitors) as part of our support network while our bodies prepare for potential pregnancy, but then compels us toward the more genetically powerful dominant males during ovulation and fertility.

The evolutionary problem of the pill is that it *disrupts* this selection cycle. Women on hormonal contraceptives do not go through the normal cycling patterns with ovulation which would lead them to choose certain immune-superior, genetically diverse (from them) males for mating, versus other males chosen for protection and nurturing. Women on OC will enter into mating relationships with the similar "kin" men and then wonder what happened to their love when they stop taking the pill to conceive and become fertile. Gals who choose their marriage partners while taking the pill report less sexual and relationship satisfaction long term and are more often the person to leave the relationship when it starts to fail a few years later. One of the most prescribed medications of our time "tells" a woman that she wants one kind of man (the coalitional male), yet when she is ready to start a family, her body instinctually realizes that he may not be the best choice to meet her biological "need" to produce the healthiest offspring. Both partners are then left in shock at their somewhat sudden disconnect.

We are just now looking at what happens to the reproductive success and children from pairings of MHC similar parents, such as those that occur while the woman is on the pill. The time it takes to conceive is greater in couples with MHC similarities. This genetic closeness appears to cause more hurdles for fertility in these couples. It also appears that miscarriage rates may be higher for these pregnancies once they are conceived. And evidence is growing that low birth weight of babies occurs more commonly with parental MHC similarity. It is very likely that the next decade will prove out the lack of wisdom in stopping pregnancy by treating women with a systemically (body-wide) active hormone such as the pill.

In providing you with this science, I am not telling you whether to use the pill or not. Surely, it has provided sexual equality for women unlike any other factor in our lifetime. But I hope you will weigh this data into your personal and marital decision making. More information and perhaps a hormonal birth control hiatus during a couple's engagement may help many of us look more fully at the partners we choose for long-term pair-bonds.

Radical Center Ruminations - There is sufficient evidence to warrant a large national clinical study to evaluate mate immune complex (MHC) similarity between women using hormonal contraceptives and their partners, and its relationship to problems with fertility, pregnancy, and offspring early childhood development.

Additionally, authors of a recent study (Gori and colleagues, September 2014) again confirmed that women on the pill show decreased attraction to men with masculine features (as markers of high genetic quality) as compared to women not taking the pill. These authors suggest, "Given the centrality of relationship satisfaction and offspring quality in (the) women and mothers, drug companies marketing hormonal contraceptives should (complete) large scale clinical trials investigating the behavioral and psychological side effects of pill use on mate choice and offspring health." Hell yes! Think of the number of couples and families impacted. We need to better understand the impact of hormonal contraceptives on us as individuals and as a species.

The Role of the Coalitional Male

For our ancestors, sexual puberty and reproduction led right off the bat to a woman seeking out that rocking stud, dominant male to father her children. But typically, these dominant men were not good providers because they were busy fighting off other men or mating with lots of ladies. After being wooed and wowed by this guy long enough to become pregnant, our great-great-grandmothers would have needed a social structure that then allowed her to raise the dominant male's baby. Looking at human historical evidence, clues in prehistoric artifacts and our closest primate relatives, it looks like most women would have raised their children in groups of other women, with input from nondominant, *coalitional* males.

These men would have been socially capable (unlike the dominant male who tended to be a loner and a "mating machine"). These men could hunt and share food. They were more stable in their social group (not having to be constantly fighting) and also likely to get a little sexual action now and then from the ladies they hung out with. The coalitional man's social functioning skills and daily proximity to groups of women would create his only chance at reproducing, unless he felt himself growing in strength and dominance to the point he wanted to knock off the alpha male.

Remember too, even if he never competed overtly with the most powerful dominant man, he was still in subtle ways competing with other coalitional males around him. The only chance coalitional men would have had of fathering children was if they were tapped for the role by the women around them. If these males had any hope of making babies, they had to remain ever vigilant and not miss any opportunity to have sex with a woman. Most men in human society, by the way, are these coalitional males. Very few males, statistically, are the dominant male. Although this alpha male gets a lot of press and many movies are made about his lonely heroism, in reality, our day-to-day lives are primarily shaped by and spent with the coalitional men around us.

Really He Isn't Just Being a Jerk

Women have asked me why men often interpret verbal and nonverbal communication from women as flirtatious and seductive even when the woman does not recall being either. In general, this mismatch in male/female interpretation is not occurring because men are jerks or because women are indiscriminately "leading on" men. It occurs because of the reproductive neurobiology that drives our subconscious mating strategies. For men, a false negative interpretation of what the cute girl said (e.g., missing a reproductive opportunity) is more costly than a false positive (e.g., perceiving the girl was hitting on him when she wasn't). So the male brain became wired to over-interpret female signals in order not to miss any possible chance to mate. This ancient male lens on the world is on display today at any bar or frat house party. And it isn't male misbehavior to hope that your text means he will get some action tonight—it's his evolutionary job.

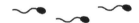

By better understanding our human mating habits and how they came to be, we hopefully can learn how to love and be in partnership with one another from *within* our natural inclinations rather than in futile opposition to them. Had I understood all of this when I was younger, perhaps I wouldn't have gone through with my wedding to Jay, even though he was a very good, talented man. I might have taken more time to understand the misgivings I was having, instead of being wooed by the "fairy tale" dress and the instinctual whispers of awesome future kids.

Chapter 5

Practice Makes Perfect - Sometimes

In 1981, after several years at Vanderbilt majoring in bio-chemistry with a minor in anthropology, I entered veterinary school at the University of Tennessee. Being the ever unusual me, I attended anatomy lab and dissected a 1,200-pound dead horse in a navy "fascinator" hat with black net veil. My professor called me "Fashion Plate" which I misheard as "Fascia Face" (fascia is the connective tissue that covers muscles), initiating my new vet school nickname.

During school I became interested in gene conservation programs for collecting and banking sperm and embryos from "heirloom" breeds of local livestock with uniquely beneficial genes around the world. For example, the N'dama cattle in Africa have evolved to be resistant to the tsetse fly. These cattle don't make much milk, so even though they were hardy survivors in the 1980s, their gene pool was dying out as farmers chose Western breeds of cattle to optimize milk production. I wanted to be involved in World Health Organization efforts to preserve gametes from diverse endangered breeds such as the N'dama. I decided that my best route to qualify for work in these conservation programs was to go practice Large Animal Medicine for a few years, then return to school for a PhD in reproductive physiology.

Throughout vet school, Jay and I continued to work to balance our personal lives and my demanding studies. We had learned how to please each other physically, but I continued to have chronic genital pain after we made love that colored our intimacy negatively during the "after glow" that usually strengthens a couple's pair-bond. Now I know that part of this chronic irritation was a result of our consistent use of lubricants during sex. What should have been helping was actually hurting. Who would have known then that vaginal lubricants would come to play such a pivotal role in my life?

Coincidentally, at the same time I was worsening my sex life at home in part by using K-Y, I also learned that it and other lubricants kill sperm. The Equine Clinic at the University of Tennessee was always busy with horses coming and going. One day, a tall bay Tennessee Walker stallion was brought in to have his semen quality tested. His wavy black mane and tail shone in the summer sun as he stepped out of the trailer. His owner led the stallion up alongside the "phantom mare" (a big ottoman couch-like contraption mounted on a pole in the air about four feet high). The owner and our clinic team waited for the stallion to mount the phantom, as if jumping on a mare, so that his semen could be collected. My job was to hold the artificial vagina (AV) and direct the stallion's penis into it. This required me to run under the stallion once he was on top of the phantom and insert his penis into the AV (an 18-inch long rubber and leather device filled with warm water, weighing about twenty pounds). To the stallion, the AV's soft inner core would feel like the inside of a mare so that he would ejaculate into it. The semen would then run into a small plastic vial attached to the end of the AV. The semen, with the sperm swimming inside it, could then be evaluated under a microscope to see whether or not the stallion was fertile.

As we worked with the stallion, our professor, Dr. John Hopkins, said, "Don't ever use any lubricant inside an artificial vagina because it will kill the sperm." He explained further: "If you use a lubricant, like K-Y, the sperm will be dead, so you can't look at them to evaluate if they are healthy, and you can't use them to artificially inseminate a mare." This comment was just a brief teaching moment for future veterinarians, but it would impact my life in a profound way. I began to wonder *why* the K-Y Jelly killed sperm and if the mechanism for this could be causing irritation or damage to other cells in the body (such as my vulvar and vaginal cells). Over the last three decades, I've been involved in many similar exams, but that first time is locked in my memory as the one that sent me on the road to inventing Pre-Seed.

After I graduated from vet school, we moved back to the Seattle area. There I literally wrote every local veterinarian in the phonebook for a job. But the reality of the market in 1984 was that very few women worked on cows, horses or other farm animals. These were "a man's job." Finally, I found a job in a mixed animal practice without a salary. Earnings were based purely on commission in the southeast Seattle clinic. This was an "If you build it, they will come" job (I hoped).

In an oddly synchronistic way, my very first case in this practice involved a lubricant emergency! Soon after I arrived at the clinic that first morning, I received a page from a large local barn. Scott, one of the top trail horses in the American Quarter Horse Association, was not able to complete his breeding to a young virgin mare. When I got to the barn, right away I could see what the problem was. Scott was very well endowed, even for a horse! His erect penis would not fit inside the little mare's vulva. I remembered Dr. Hopkins' "lubricants kill sperm" lecture, so we couldn't use K-Y. I asked Frank, the owner of the barn, "Do you guys have any Vaseline in your bathroom?"

Frank nodded, went to his bathroom at the house and brought the jar back to me. I coated Vaseline over any male and female surfaces involved in the breeding then watched nervously as Frank guided Scott, with his full erection, back up to the mare. Scott mounted the mare in a powerful lunge and then slid right inside her vulva.

I was so excited I literally jumped up and down, clapping my hands in victory. It had worked! I did it! Here had been my first healthcare problem that I had used *my* knowledge to solve. Years later I would learn that Vaseline also has a mildly toxic effect on sperm, but in this case the stars all aligned, and our girl got pregnant. At twenty-four years of age I had learned that although lubricants can be bad for sperm, sometimes they are just plain necessary to fit a (large) round peg in a (sort of) square hole.

Over the next few years, as I worked 80 or more hours a week in my practice, Jay and I let our enjoyment of each other continue to fade. Although we were able to talk together as friends when we had time, the first clue of our marital distress came in a growing lack of fulfillment in our sex lives. We both had high sex drives, so we continued making love as schedules allowed, but this became more about the release of orgasm as numerous factors kept us from becoming "partners in pleasure" and growing together in our sexual satisfaction.

Research shows that couples such as us who have a rough start on their sexual compatibility in the first years of marriage have a higher rate of marriage failure. Bad sex isn't insurmountable, but the pair-bond isn't adequately supported when there is no oxytocin release in the partners, such as good lovemaking can bring. And equally important, it is likely that the couple will not develop a lexicon for sharing what they want sexually to create together a reassuring and uplifting *sexual script*. A sexual script allows us to make love as a couple in a predictable way, knowing what the other wants and needs...and when. These scripts keep us from having to always discuss or guess what the next move is, and it can decrease conflict for the couple during and around sex.

For my twenty-something self, suffering from chronic post-coital irritation (a condition called *provoked vestibulodynia* that I will discuss more later), the burning, raw pain I felt after lovemaking became part of our sexual script. This was not what either one of us wanted, or expected, from intimacy. Blame and disappointment often seemed to follow. If two people do not find deeper intimacy through sex, it can instead lead to loneliness and exacerbate marital flaws. Allowing our love life to lack intensity or fun and failing to dedicate the time to seek professional help to deal with my chronic pain condition were both symptoms and causes of our failing marriage.

I have interacted with many other couples since then who also want to succeed in their marriages yet don't know enough about their sexuality and its impact on romance and marriage to help them reach their goal. Couples normally go through waves of sexual fulfillment. Job stress, trying to conceive, pregnancy, injury, military deployments, menopause and andropause, failing bodies, mental illness, loneliness, fights and "I hate you" times all can impact our sexual enjoyment of each other. To help couples during the good times and the bad times, I have developed some "Gourmet Sex" ideas. Our hormones and blood chemistry are utterly linked with sexuality, so "closer-via-sex" is a primary way to ensure closeness in other aspects of intimacy and marriage.

Gourmet Sex - Spice It Up!

Please beware, this section is X-rated. If this kind of graphic and honest sex talk feels uncomfortable, skip ahead in the book then wander back here when you feel comfortable. DH in these sex tips is short for "Darling Husband." Of course, your DH can be any man who cares about your sexual pleasure.

All of the sex positions and activities in this chapter can be enhanced with Pre-Seed lubricant. When the right amount of Pre-Seed is applied, your organs feel slippery and natural ("slippery when wet"), not sticky or tacky. Importantly, Pre-Seed doesn't taste bad, so using *it doesn't interfere with great oral sex.* Also, because it doesn't have silicone in it, Pre-Seed washes off easily. Remember that the "right amount" of the lubricant depends on what specific sex act you are engaging in. If your Pre-Seed application dries out too fast, you didn't use *enough* to saturate the skin and then to lubricate. If, on the other hand, the organs become too slippery (he may say he feels "numb"), stop, wipe everybody off with the sheet or a washcloth and go on with sex...then use less next time. Because Pre-Seed is applied inside with a vaginal applicator, it feels more natural and lasts longer than other lubricants. After applying Pre-Seed during washing up or getting ready for sex, you can walk around or even go to the bathroom. It will stay deep inside coating the vaginal walls providing lubrication for later.

For everyday sex (not babymaking), usually only one to two grams are needed when placed deep inside the woman, so the 40 gm tube can last a long time. If you are trying to conceive, NEVER wash or reuse the applicator (soaps and water kill sperm). If you need extra vaginal applicators, they can be purchased online at *TrulyConceivable.com*. Personally, since I am not trying to conceive, I wash the applicators with warm water and soap and let them dry on a clean towel, using them several times before discarding. I use Pre-Seed almost every time we make love because I love the slippery feeling during foreplay as well as intercourse itself. For couples who like using a silicone lubricant, the Replens® Silky Smooth is an excellent product.

Find Your Best Body Image Lingerie

Most of us gals have some body image issues when naked or in lingerie. This makes sex problematic for our guys—we don't want them looking at anyone else's body, but, simultaneously, we won't show them ours. Yet males are hard-wired for sex through not just the penis but also the visual cortex. I have found that the best lingerie for those times when you feel self-conscious, but still want great sex, is a crotchless and cupless teddy. Trust me, even if you don't normally do "skank," guys LOVE this! And it covers everything you don't want showing (sagging tummy, love muffins) but shows "just the facts" (tits, pussy and ass). Plus you will look perfect in it whether you have small breasts or large. I like item #4100 Tres Sexy by Oh La La Cheri. It fits most people, large or small, and it isn't expensive. Try it and once you have it on…don't act shy…just be brazen.

Titty Sex

For this one, ladies, prop yourself up with pillows behind you so that you are sitting against the headboard with your legs spread out. Have DH kneel between your legs so that you have good access to his genitals. Put a lot of lubricant on your hand then on his cock. Next wrap your hand around his shaft and slide your hand up and down—all the way to the base and then up and over the tip. Meanwhile, use your thumb to keep pressure on the ridge on the underside of his penis, flicking your thumb occasionally over the end as you reach the top. Use the other hand to caress his balls or to slide a lubricated finger along his backside, and even inside him.

As he gets more excited, let him squeeze your tits together from each side. Then he can thrust his cock in between them. You can help him keep your breasts squeezed together by using your upper arms to smoosh them together. Keep your hand below your breasts wrapped around his penis so that he continues having firm pressure on his cock as he thrusts up and down. This way even if you have smaller breasts, he still gets the pressure needed to orgasm—and a great visual of the head of his penis sliding up and down between them.

For us gals, this position is probably the least labor intensive, and it works any time you don't want anyone messing around "down there," such as postpartum or when you have "female" issues related to menses. Of course, this position doesn't mean you don't get to orgasm. If you want an orgasm, have him take care of you first and then switch to this position.

Doggy Style With Added Hand Pressure

This is a great position if you want to spice up sex in general, want to add variety to trying-to-conceive sex, are pregnant or just feel "fat conscious." It is also great if you have something going on in your life that impedes super deep penetration (e.g., post-surgery or endometriosis). The added hand pressure on DH in this position is great for us older gals who have had kids and feel a bit "loose" back there.

Lube up by putting Pre-Seed *inside* the vagina with the provided applicator while you wash up, so the slip and slide lasts through the stroking of intercourse. Kneel on the bed, have DH enter vaginally from behind, and then turn your head and drop your shoulders and rest your cheek on the bed. Reach your right hand back between your legs and wrap your hand over your vulva (as if you were cupping yourself), making a peace sign in front of your vulva. DH should then be thrusting in and out of your vagina with your fingers squeezing against him on either side. By squeezing your fingers together as hard as you can against his cock, your "peace sign fingers" increase pressure on him as he thrusts. Having your fingers between your vulva and his cock also limits how deep he is thrusting so that you can pull away a bit if it is getting too deep.

Side Sex with Added Pressure

This position works well for injured people or those wanting more mellow sex. It is also a great TTC position. It can even be modified to limit penetration depth if you are recovering from surgery (such as a hysterectomy) or have deep pain during intercourse.

Again, lube up with Pre-Seed by applying it inside the vagina with the applicator. This position requires *a lot* of lubrication. Lie down facing each other on the bed (ladies, we will say you are on your right side). Drape your left leg over DH's thighs and have him enter you vaginally. Reach your left hand around behind your left thigh and buttocks so you can feel DH's cock going in and out of your vulva. Use your fingers to push him down and into you while he thrusts in and out so that he is feeling the firm pressure of your fingers pushing against him, as well as your moist vagina as he moves in and out. You really can't push too firmly on him in this position— more firmly is good! And for this position to work, the downward pressure on his penis needs to be constant until he comes. Depending on the angle, you may feel that your fingers are pushing him straight into you. A bonus to this is the added hand pressure and stimulation if DH has been drinking or if he has been taking antidepressants, either of which can make him slow to come.

Lady on Top

Having the women on top has been shown in studies to improve female orgasm rates. It is also good if DH has problems with not lasting as long as you need him erect. As you do this position, remember that the more Pre-Seed you use, the more slippery his cock will be and the less sensation he will feel so play around with amounts to see if you can help him last longer. You can get great stimulation and also make him last longer by grinding or rocking back and forth, rather than going up and down on his shaft. If deep penetration isn't feeling good to you (e.g., time of the month or endometriosis), instead of sitting up on him where he can kiss and caress your breasts, lie down across his stomach while he is in you and keep kissing each other so that you control the depth you slide back and onto his penis. This way, you control the amount of penetration, making it feel the most comfortable for you.

Oral Sex Without Swallowing

I really enjoy the sensations of oral sex, but sometimes I am just not in the mood to swallow. To give a great BJ without swallowing, put a tablespoon of Pre-Seed in your hand and lube him up. For added eye candy for DH, kneel on all fours in front of him as he kneels on the bed. This way he can play with your ass and pussy by reaching behind you from the top. This is not a position for the physically unfit, so an easier, more passive way to give a guy good oral sex is to have him sit on the edge of the bed and you kneel or sit in front of him.

Either way you choose, lube his cock up super well then start with a nice firm hand job, encircling him firmly with your whole hand and placing your thumb on the ridge on the underside of his penis. Remember to stroke the thumb up and down and sometimes flick it over the tip of his penis as you stroke up. Ask him to grab your head and pull you to him when he is ready for a switch from hand to oral action. Then be sure to keep a vigorous hand job going even while you suck on him...but sometimes stop your hand to take him deeply in your mouth. During this phase of the BJ, wrap your lips around DH's parts. Use your other hand to play with his balls and, if you want, his ass. Keep your hand right next to your lips so it is a continuous sensation for him. Be sure to cup your lips around your teeth slightly while doing this. As he gets closer to orgasm, thrust your tongue out long and soft (think Maori warrior tongue) so that as he slides in and out, he will have a continuous sensation between your hands, your warm soft tongue and your firmer, tighter upper lip.

The benefit of the lubricant is that you can keep slippery wet pressure on him through a combination of hand and mouth. In fact, as he gets closer to coming, increase the hand stroke length so that your hand comes all the way up over the tip of his penis and your upper lip comes off him for a second (but your hand keeps him pulled against your flat broad tongue). When he comes, open your mouth very wide and keep the hand pressure on tight, pulling him against your tongue the whole time. If you wish, just let everything that "comes" fall back out of your mouth onto your hand and/or the bed or cloth you have ready. He won't mind the switch up if it means more oral sex. He wants the oral sex!

And guys, if you are done having kids, think about getting a vasectomy. This will decrease ejaculate volume and make oral sex more common in your house.

Fabulous Oral Sex for Her

Often, men hyperfocus on the exterior glans of the clitoris during foreplay and oral sex, which can make women irritated and sore. This kind of intense contact makes me want to slap DH! Also, for smoother sailing, guys take a minute to shave off that five o'clock shadow. Bristly hairs around the mouth can be a real turn off if they start scratching or poking private parts. To perfect oral sex on the ladies, I highly recommend Ian Kerner's *She Comes First*. Dr. Kerner teaches a combination of "movement and stillness" as modified here. His tongue (or hers if you are a lesbian couple) should be flat and soft (think Maori warrior again). When he first approaches, you can be lying on your back with knees bent. Coach DH to press his flat tongue softly against your vulvar opening (not clitoral head), hold for a moment; and then break the contact fully.

Now, men, kiss her vulva and clitoral area all around in five to ten soft pressing kisses, ending with a flat tongue pressed for five seconds against the head of her clitoris. Then lick slowly from the top of her vaginal opening to the bottom ten times in a slow steady rhythm. This protects her clitoral head from a strong, potentially irritating "cross grain" stroke that occurs if you lick repeatedly against this area.

Next step—as she becomes excited, initially avoid the head of the clitoris. Instead, use a small halfway lick from the bottom to the mid vulva, focusing on the inner labia for a series of five unrushed licks, then lick all the way up the full vulva and over the clit head, pressing the tip of your tongue softly over the clitoral head for five seconds on the sixth stroke.

Now go back to the halfway licks, increasing by one each time with the "head bath" at the end of each repetition. Repeat this ten to twenty times. Keep a steady rhythm while you are doing this. As your woman gets close to orgasm, follow her lead. When she gives you verbal cues and lifts her hips toward you, things are going well!

Although it may feel weird to count in your mind while doing this, guys, the counting is actually very helpful to pleasuring your woman. The counting slows you down and makes you be more gentle with your woman's body and thus more able to give her the gift of a great orgasm.

The biggest mistakes men make in cunnilingus are 1) rushing and 2) too much constant or firm contact of tongue on the clitoral head. Remember there is a great big clitoris for you to stimulate and enjoy!

What I Didn't Know

Despite a struggling marriage, some of my fondest memories are from my time in general veterinary practice—watching a frisky foal nurse from its mom, with Mount Rainier in glorious view over the barn roof, or delivering newborn lambs in cozy stalls filled with straw on snowy winter days. I loved these parts of practice. But the long hours, the constant on-call, the blurred lines between "friends" and clients (and resulting lack of private time) and the need to charge people for what I did (even when things didn't turn out as we hoped and an animal died) were all difficult and stressful for me. I started thinking more about when I would head back to school for that PhD in reproductive physiology and as our marriage continued to fade, I wondered if that move would be something that included Jay or not.

Through these years, intimacy and chronic urinary tract infections (UTIs) continued to be a source of pain even when we weren't having sex. This irritation was likely exacerbated by the K-Y we often used during lovemaking and certainly by the birth control pills I was taking to avoid an unplanned pregnancy. The tight jeans I wore and the long miles I sat driving in the car to the far-flung farms of western Washington also made things worse. But I had no idea that any of these could cause the pelvic pain symptoms I was experiencing. We made love several times a week, but afterwards I always felt rawness that would last a day or two...so in my mind the pain was from the sex. None of my doctors told me that birth control pills are highly associated with the development of painful sex, vaginal dryness and chronic UTIs in women. Nor did the doctors explain how I could successfully manage the painful intercourse. I didn't know that almost half of all women will have painful intercourse at some time in their lives and that there were solutions for women like me. Specifically, I would learn later that I had *provoked vestibulodynia* (PVD) or *vulvodynia*, a chronic pain condition affecting about 20% of women. This condition caused the relentless burning and irritation I experienced not just right after sex but also for hours and days afterwards. Even walking, sitting down and wearing certain clothes could feel unbearable.

Physicians were just beginning in the late 1980s to understand this condition. Medicine had been dominated by men over the past centuries and women with PVD were thought to just not like "doing their duty" in the marriage bed. As more women came into the field, many who had experienced PVD themselves were able to better shed light into this condition, as well as look for better answers to managing and mitigating it. Since that time, science has shown that the pill can be a risk factor for developing *lifelong* PVD and that some lubricants can also make it worse.

Genital Pain - Not All in Her Head

Genital pain is relatively common in women, with 46% reporting pain during intercourse (*dyspareunia*) at some time in life and *one in four* women suffering at some point from the chronic burning rawness of PVD. The "*vestibule*" is the genital area between the labia minora of the vulva and the urethra in women. It is the tissue that women see if they spread the lips of their vulva open and look inside themselves with a mirror. The chronic pain of PVD affects both this area and the outer vulvar lips. More than 90% of women with PVD will have pain for over a year, with *seven years* being the average length of suffering. The incidence of onset is highest among women 18-25 years old, the age I was when it happened to me.

Over 60% of women with the condition cannot have sex without pain. Like I did, they also experience nonsexual pain throughout the day, pain that compromises their quality of life, sometimes even leading to suicide. Shockingly, a recent Harvard study found that most women with PVD sought professional advice from *three or more physicians, with 40% of these women incorrectly diagnosed even after their third medical opinion*!

The genital pain and redness of PVD can be provoked by hormone changes, prolonged sitting and by contact with many different common items, such as saliva, semen, vibrators, tight clothes and any number of feminine hygiene products including lubricants. Women with PVD have pressure receptors in the skin that become over stimulated from chronic "allergy-like" irritation, thus triggering pain responses in the brain. *A potential link between the use of oral contraceptives and development of PVD has been shown in the last decade.* For me, this link would have been very important to know at the time as I had my worst PVD while on the pill.

Determining What Kind of Pain Women Have During Sex

Dyspareunia, or painful intercourse, is pain felt during penetration or thrusting, specifically during sex (it does not necessarily have the residual "chemical burning" feeling of PVD). It can be caused by a number of factors, including PVD. Other causes are listed below:

- *Thinning of the vaginal wall (atrophic vaginitis)* as happens in 40% of menopausal women, in women on low-dose contraceptives and in women following cancer therapy.

- *Interstitial Cystitis/Painful Bladder Syndrome (IC/PBS)* is a chronic disease known for bladder pain and increased urinary urgency and frequency. It is thought to be due to a chemical deficiency of the cells lining the bladder. Additionally, one third of women with IC/PBS also have PVD (sorry for all the acronyms—but, in short, everything hurts on these gals!)

- *Pelvic Floor Hypertonus* (Vaginismis) is a chronic spasm of the muscle of the pelvic floor. It can occur on its own or secondarily as a result of trauma, or pelvic cancer treatment. Because there is no conscious control over these muscle spasms, it feels similar to blinking your eye closed when someone tries to touch it, only it is the vagina that reactively closes.

- *Vulvar Dermatologic Conditions (including contact allergies or lichen sclerosis or autoimmune diseases)* are conditions that require disease-specific management.

- *Endometriosis* is the most common cause of deep pelvic pain in women. Treatment requires medical or surgical management as well as physician expertise with the syndrome.

Because these conditions are so consistently incorrectly diagnosed and treated, get a second opinion if you are diagnosed with one of them. Your doctor should understand if you want to seek this out. Some women spend years with an incorrect diagnosis and therapy, and the chronic pain condition can take a toll on couples and families.

Optimize Your Care Provider's Ability to Help You

If you are feeling pain in your pelvic region, you can take proactive steps to increase the likelihood of a correct diagnosis, sooner rather than later. Get a small writing journal you keep near your bed and follow these steps.

- Write down the dates of any significant events that have happened to you involving this area (e.g., surgeries, childbirth, abortions, cancer therapy).

- Be sure to indicate whether you have always had the pain or if it has only been present at particular times in your life.

- Write down issues about your health in general (e.g., dandruff, psoriasis, dry eyes, mental health treatment, thyroid problems, asthma and diabetes).

- Write down every day for a month exactly what made your pain worse or better: What clothes did you wear? Did you sit or exercise? Did you have sex? What did you eat more or less of? What products did you use near your vagina?

- If you had pain during sex, write down what positions you used and at what point during sex it hurt (foreplay, penetration, thrusting, orgasm and/or afterwards). Then focus on your body and "feel" the pain again to use descriptive words to write down what happened and how you felt. For example, some women might say:

  - ✔ "I have an *aching pain* when he thrusts deeply."

  - ✔ "I feel a *burning pain* when he penetrates."

  - ✔ "There is a *sharp pain* when he touches my clitoris."

  - ✔ "I have an *uncomfortable, tingling pain* after intercourse."

- If you feel sore outside of sex, write down when you feel this, such as sitting at work, driving in the car, after wiping on the toilet, when wearing pants or when it is hot out.

- Be sure to write down where you are in your menstrual cycle when the pain occurs. Also include when you had your period and if you have any infections or weird smells or discharges.

Type this all up in an organized fashion and hand it to the nurse when you go see a doctor for your problems. It will revolutionize the quality of care you get. Most of us haven't thought about these things carefully and therefore can't even begin to articulate them to a physician or nurse.

Tips for Managing Vulvar Pain Conditions

As I have learned for myself and by assisting other women and couples, here are some of my tips for managing vulvar pain.

Clothes matter!

I never wear tight jeans or any pants with uncomfortable seams over my "bits." When I shop for clothes, I reach inside every pair of pants to feel the seams. I like gusseted pants, such as those by Kuhl, but I usually just wear long jersey skirts. I think people wonder if I am Amish, but I don't care. I even farm in these skirts!

Finding the right *underwear* has also been the "Holy Grail" of my life. Underwear makers have cheapened the products for girls and women so that almost all have seams in the wrong places. For me, cotton is bad, even though most doctors and even the National Institutes of Health will tell you to wear cotton (based on NO scientific data). But beware, cotton holds in wetness from urine and vaginal secretions. I can wear Patagonia's® Barely underwear made from polyester and Spandex. This product dries quickly and has no seam.

In any case, remember that wearing nothing at night is important in order for your private parts to air out.

Use Only Truly Nonirritating Soaps on Your Private Parts

Even if a product says it is "mild," usually those with glycerin, glycerol or propylene glycol (even baby shampoos) may have an ion content that is too high for you. This can cause irritation of the vulva. My favorite wash is Organix® Soothing Teatree Peppermint Body Wash. It never causes me any irritation.

Use Pre-Seed to Lubricate for Sex

Pre-Seed has the same salt concentration as body fluids. Had I not suffered from "very finicky parts" myself, I may not have developed such a mild Pre-Seed formula. As you will learn later, I tested all the different Pre-Seed prototypes on myself. If they caused me any irritation at all, the recipe was scrapped; finally we developed a formula that was mild enough to make babies *and* didn't cause me any irritation, even with daily use.

Shave It All Off

Shaving everything off, including those parts of him that go inside the woman can make a positive difference in keeping irritation to a minimum. We keep Venus® razors with the gel strip for a smooth glide in the shower. It takes one minute to whisk things clean each day. Men grow more hair along the length of the penis as they age; this hair can cause irritation, especially for women who are going through thinning of their genital tissue during menopause. So, men, I know some of you will balk at shaving the hair off your penis, but seriously, when you are by yourself, take a look at the rough, curly pubic hairs growing up your erect shaft (yes, do this when you have a hard on). You'll understand that they can irritate your partner's vagina if she has genital pain issues.

Use Medications Wisely

Hormone replacement therapy can be *critical* for lessening symptoms after menopause and, in younger women, for assisting with abnormal cycle activity such as postpartum or with premature ovarian failure. I use a Vivelle® patch, testosterone injections, and Vagifem® inter-vaginal tabs to keep my parts healthy.

If you suffer from PVD or dyspareunia, hormonal contraceptives such as pills, shots and rings may not be good because some have been shown to decrease arousal and increase pain at intercourse. You might want to talk to your doctor about an IUD (which does not harm libido) or think about using carefully executed Fertility Awareness-based Methods (FAMs) as detailed in Toni Weschler's *Taking Charge of Your Fertility.*

Many times pelvic pain sufferers are put on SSRI antidepressants, but these can decrease arousal fluids, libido and orgasm response and make intercourse last longer, which is NOT what you want. If you need antidepressants, talk to your doctor about other options that may not cause some of these symptoms. Especially in women with chronic diseases, such as Multiple Sclerosis and bipolar disease, new studies suggest that the negative effects of SSRIs on sexuality make them a poor choice.

Try a Bidet

A special toilet seat that washes the woman's vulvar region and backside with water can limit PVD irritation. Constant wiping with toilet paper or wet wipes can cause microabrasions that residual urine may further irritate. I started using a bidet, and it greatly decreased my symptoms. An inexpensive option to try for yourself is available at Costco®. If you try this, let me know if it makes a difference for you. I would like to write a grant to research the use of bidets for PVD patients.

Don't Forget Your Man

Male partners of women with dyspareunia experience less sexual fulfillment and more erectile dysfunction than men in couples not dealing with this condition. Men don't want to cause pain in their women and may feel helpless. At the same time, sexual communication between partners coping with dyspareunia is often significantly poorer as these women struggle with how often to mention their pain and what triggers it. To keep things spicy for him, occasionally try some of my previous Gourmet Sex Tips. Remember, it isn't his fault you have PVD—so treat him with patience and compassion, just as you want for yourself. Both you and your partner should remember that having PVD or dyspareunia doesn't mean you don't like sex or that either partner is "bad" at sex.

PVD and related pelvic diseases are medical conditions that interfere with what should be enjoyable human behavior. You live with this condition and based on the research you are doing, you may initially know more than your regular doctor. Keep looking for the doctor who knows more than you, such as doctors who belong to the National Vulvodynia Association (*nva.org*), British Society for the Study of Vulval Disease (*bssvd.org*), and the International Society for Sexual Medicine (*issm.info*). *When Sex Hurts: A Woman's Guide to Banishing Sexual Pain,* written by Dr. Andrew Goldstein (and others), is a good lay reference book. Also recommended is the book *Sex Without Pain: A Self-Treatment Guide To The Sex Life*

You Deserve written by Dr. Heather Jeffcoat, a physical therapist with countless successes in treating pain of this type. Women with vaginismus, overactive pelvic floor, painful intercourse, vulvodynia, vulvar vestibulitis, vestibulodynia, dyspareunia, and interstitial cystitis can benefit from her unique, easy to follow program.

Radical Center Ruminations - Six million Americans currently experience ongoing debilitating genital pain from provoked vestibulodynia—more than the 4.5 million Americans wearing orthodontics! Only 2% of women with PVD are accurately diagnosed when they first go to the doctor. Diagnosis is poor in some part because anything that happens down there "must" be a yeast infection. Additionally, evidenced-based medical approaches are lacking because of poor research funding for a disease that impacts so many people. Our daughters (and therefore the men they have sex with) deserve better.

If you are a PVD sufferer or spouse, share your story with your state and federal representatives and ask him or her to start treating and funding it like a real disease and not just a "woman thing." Let's start with having a study on the best type of underwear to decrease PVD symptoms.

Overtime, I learned that lots of small changes helped me manage my sensitive "down under," as well as eventually taking more radical steps, such as stopping oral contraceptives. The chronic pain I experienced in my relationship with Jay went on for years without appropriate diagnosis or treatment, coloring many aspects of our lives. Of course, beyond the PVD, we also had other marital issues as our lives led us in different directions towards new goals and away from each other.

Chapter 6

Struggling To Relate

In 1986, I had the opportunity to go to India to lecture at veterinary colleges about the use of embryo transfer and artificial insemination for conserving local cattle breeds. I was finally on my way to saving endangered livestock species! But as much as I was mentoring the people in India, I was actually learning more from them in return. Each day I met people who were living lives that were very different from mine but who were finding meaning and happiness even as they struggled with far fewer opportunities than most Americans. I began to understand that my worldview was too narrow and that life and relationships were much more complex than I had been taught or had realized. With a growing mixture of fear and hope, I knew it was time to move on from where I was in my personal life, both at home and at work.

When Jay and I returned home, we discussed the fact that our worlds were drifting apart and that we were headed in opposite directions. He would go on to become a pastor; I would go on to invent a sex lubricant! We stayed married a bit longer but lived separate lives as we tried to figure out the logistics of a divorce. It was clear that Jay and I were not going to be successful in mating for life.

Are Humans Monogamous?

Although mating for life is lifted up as the ideal form for romantic relationships, many of us can't seem to make it work. And whenever the majority cannot abide by a cultural "should," it is likely that these expectations are misaligned with who we are as human beings at a *biological and instinctual* level. Although monogamy is perceived as a "natural" state in Western society, its origins in human culture are relatively new (even people in the Bible were not monogamous), and its execution is plagued by societal contradictions. Interestingly, something as basic as our dictionary definition shows our ambivalence toward what we expect from monogamy. The *archaic* definition (at *merriam-webster.com*) is "the practice of marrying only once during a lifetime." A newer definition is "the state or custom of being married to only one person at a time." And the most recent definition is "the condition or practice of having a single mate during a period of time." Under the latter, I suppose a one-night stand could be considered monogamous, if the "period of time" is 12 hours!

Usually when we think or talk about monogamy within our relationships, we are really referring to marriage fidelity. Many of us expect our partners to be sexually faithful to us. But let's look at how we *actually* live according to the scientific data.

In fact, only a quarter of Americans have only had one lifetime sexual partner, and these folks are mainly from an older generation that may yet take on other partners as they age and/or their spouse dies. Additionally, many people have at least one extra-marital interaction. According to the latest research, rates of at least one incident of infidelity are 30-50% for married men and 20-40% for women. Taken together, the total lifetime chance that at least one partner has had sex outside of the couple is as high as 75%!

Part of our confused, contradictory approach to marriage and monogamy comes from our inability as a society to look honestly at these institutions so that we can have private and public conversations grounded in facts. For example, Americans who are the most religiously conservative (such as Jay and I were) are actually the most at risk of divorce. This may seem counterintuitive, but it has been shown to be true in numerous studies (e.g., Glass and Levchak, 2014).

Additionally, many of us in Hometown, America may not realize just how much change is occurring in our institutions of marriage and family, as detailed in a recent 2012 presidential report *The State of Our Unions: Marriage in America*. In particular, there is a "striking exodus" from marriage among high school-educated young people (i.e., those who have not gone to college). Men and women from this group often move in together and have children. But couples that live together and have a child are twice as likely as married couples to break up before that child turns twelve. This group then often enters into serial "monogamous" partnerships that are becoming the new normal for the demographic. Or as the report quotes, "Americans are stepping 'on and off the carousel of intimate relationships' increasingly rapidly." The new dictionary definition of monogamy is simply keeping pace with how we are living. We are with one person for as long as we are with them.

These changes in cohabitation and intimate relationships are changing our family structure too. In the 1980s, only 13% of children of moderately-educated mothers were born outside of marriage, but by the late 2000s, this figure rose to a striking 44%! And more than half of births in the U.S. today among women under 30 occur outside of marriage. Sometimes we are prone to think that all these out-of-wedlock births are "other" people, but the average American woman bearing a child outside of marriage now is a twenty-something white woman with a high school degree.

Even for those of us who are getting married, things have changed in a generation. We live together before we get married, and we don't stay married. Over 60% of first marriages are now preceded by the couple living together. And for first marriages, about 50% are likely to end in divorce. While some recent press has suggested that divorce rates are declining, a couple has to be married in order for divorce to occur. With a decline of more than 50% in annual marriage rates for women between 1970 and 2010, it is easy to see that how we quantify "successful" and "unsuccessful" relationships is in a time of tremendous flux. Since contraceptives have allowed us to have sex without the risk of pregnancy and parenthood, monogamy (in terms of mating for life) has become much less prevalent. The average number of lifetime sex partners has increased for Americans between the ages of 30 and 44 to eight for men and four for women. Likely these numbers will continue to increase as the upcoming generation of teens are having sex younger and with more partners at an earlier age.

So while we hold to an image of ourselves as a monogamous species, science from the past and present suggests we are *not,* or at best, we only are sometimes. But let's keep our actual goals at the forefront in this discussion. Most of us want to have fulfilling relationships and a stable environment for our children. If we can better understand why relationships fail, perhaps we can give ourselves the best chance of keeping our valued partnerships alive and healthy. One of the key factors in this quest is sex. Sexual fulfillment and sexual satisfaction are highly correlated to overall relationship satisfaction for both men and women. People in sexually satisfying relationships are statistically more likely to remain sexually faithful. People who aren't sexually fulfilled (in terms of both quality and quantity) will be some of the first to the exit door during tough times, even if it is just sneaking out the back door for a quickie elsewhere.

The reasons that people maintain sexual fidelity in their marriages are multifaceted. Just like everything else human, part of our fidelity can be predisposed by a genetic influence. Some people have genes that support monogamy and others do not. People without the monogamy gene don't all cheat, but given the same set of circumstances, they are less likely to stay faithful than people with a monogamous genetic makeup. Of course, genes don't control us: they do not necessarily determine one's destiny. But nonmonogamy genes also relate to other genes that seek adventure and high risk. As a society we need both the "Leavers"—those that set sail for adventure and the unknown—and the "Doers"—those that keep the day-to-day going. How we see ourselves on this continuum may help us look more honestly at who we are individually and sexually.

In addition to genes, sexual satisfaction for one or both partners can impact fidelity. People probably already know that men who are not sexually satisfied are at risk of cheating. You might not know though that research also shows that a lack of desire for sex by women is a leading reason women feel worried about the future of their marriage and therefore seek marriage or sex therapy. Up to 43% of American women suffer from some form of sexual dysfunction in their marriages. The overwhelmingly most common problem is low desire in the female partner that becomes significant enough to cause the couple distress.

A recent *Family Circle* survey found that 32% of mothers had gone "a few years" without having sex! What does sexual fidelity mean for the partners of these women? If couples aren't together for sex, what are they together for? And when will one (or both) of them want out so that they can feel sexual desire again? We absolutely have to work at sexual health and quality if we are to help our marriages survive because when either partner has low sexual desire for many months, a marriage is at risk. The constancy of low sexual desire must be dealt with so that the sexual, physical, psychological, emotional and spiritual connection between the two married people will not gradually dissolve. Sex is that important, especially for people under 60, because it is a primary way that pair-bonds stay stable throughout the stresses of everyday life (e.g., raising kids, working and dealing with aging parents). Sex releases chemicals that the brain needs in order to maintain the pair-bond.

What We Know Can Help Us - The Human Pair-Bond

The mating systems that have helped humans for thousands of years choose partners for procreation and sexuality differ from *marriage systems* (our culturally ascribed methods of partner formation). To complicate matters further, these two systems may differ from a third: *social partnering systems* (how we actually raise our kids and pay the bills). Several factors make these three unique systems more complex in modern society as compared to other times in human history. Most importantly we need to remember that up until the 1800s the average human life expectancy was less than 30 years old. Additionally, our offspring functioned as adults soon after puberty in their early teens. So the overall length of time people negotiated partnerships and parenting systems was far shorter than it is now.

To look at all this we need to view the "pair-bond" through the lens of human history. For much of our existence, the primal goal of women and men was to reproduce. Thus, *pair-bonding* described two people who desired each other enough to have sex as often as it took for the woman to conceive. As we have discussed, the dominant male would mate with the females that sought him out. After a female became pregnant, the relationships that supported her and raised her children were the tribe and extended family, not the dominant male. Thus, "'til pregnancy do us part" was the norm for mating pairs.

Since the rise of agriculture 10,000 or so years ago, as populations increased and social complexity, land ownership and methods of procuring food changed, polygamous pair-bonding extended the length of time for male-female interactions, with one man and his wives often forming a mating, marriage and social partnering unit through their lifetime, or until the man threw a woman and her kids out.

I want to take a moment to reiterate the profound impact the rise of agriculture has had on human social systems. Prior to this, tribes of humans foraged and hunted. Because there was no ownership of property, it did not really matter who fathered the children (other than from an evolutionary, "high quality gene" standpoint). Sex was as natural as what we see in the barnyard. Social groupings of women and coalitional males lived together and looked out for each other. Dominant males had their harem of fertile women that they mated with and guarded from other male competitors. But overall, women controlled who they mated with and when. Once humans stopped long enough to plant crops and accumulate property, social interactions became more complex as the developing systems for passing down land and wealth required certainty in paternity and greater control of female sexuality. Still this time of recorded human history is really only a fraction of our human existence—a fraction that is already passing away as our culture evolves yet again into the future.

Approximately 80% of all societies throughout the anthropologic record (recorded human history) permitted men to marry multiple wives (only 4% allowed for multiple husbands). The ability to support multiple wives was associated with status and wealth (as it still is in some cultures). However, excess males, being as much as 60% of men, did not have access to mates in these cultures, which was "great" for waging war but bad for social stability, as discussed below.

Cultural anthropology shows a new pair-bond experiment came along in the past 4,000 years—specifically that of *monogamy*. At first, monogamy was only an option, not a requirement. In the last 500 years, however, one-on-one love relationships have become more highly valued for their potential to stabilize societies and thus have been enacted into law in many countries. Decreasing the pool of unmarried men through enforced monogamy is good for social stability: It decreases crime. It can also improve commerce, innovation and social mobility. Studies have shown that the adoption of monogamy in a country leads to GDP increases as men focus on productivity rather than finding multiple wives. Lower competition between males means almost all men can find a mate and the society as a whole is more stable. Monogamous marriage is also helpful to women in many ways: it increases the women's age at marriage, decreases spousal age gaps (decreasing the practice of older men marrying young brides) and can decrease gender economic inequality. Monogamy (in the *archaic* meaning of "one mate for life") is also of course the best way to contain sexually transmitted diseases. There is a lot going for monogamy. But…

It is crucial to remember that humans mate much more based on our DNA and hormone guidance than on any words or vows in our heads. Marriage systems are defined by culture and religion, and they differ across regions. Our marriage systems don't always line up with our evolved mating strategies and our deep psyches. Human mating systems are hundreds of thousands of years old, whereas our marriage systems have been around for less than 2% of human history, and even within this short period have been ever changing. No wonder we get confused! And to further complicate matters, we are in a time of increasingly rapid transition. Although many men strayed from their monogamous pair-bonds during past generations, the marriages (especially if children were born) generally remained intact even though papa was "stepping out." The last 50 years has fundamentally altered our perception and practice of the human pair-bond as divorce, birth control and the economic independence of women have ushered in a true social revolution.

No longer do religion and culture necessarily keep monogamous marriages together. And legal constructs (such as no-fault divorce) have also evolved to mirror who many, if not most of us, truly are—nonmonogamous humans who do not necessarily mate for life.

Even though we are no longer "required" to be monogamous (e.g., we can have sex without having babies; we can divorce an ill-suited partner; and we can all earn our own money), many of us still choose this path. And there are still excellent reasons for choosing monogamy. Nonetheless, keeping a marriage alive takes work and vigilance, so if your goal is to stay married to your current partner, it can be helpful to know about certain "triggers" for infidelity. Research shows that these high-risk times can more commonly move one member of a couple from being content in a monogamous relationship to the cheater/cheated column. If these situations exist in your life and marriage, be conscious of each other and your true goals. If you want to stay married, recognize these situations and proactively work on your marriage...while it is still there.

1) Pregnancy and the birth of a new child are high-risk times for men to step out. As the male in the pair-bond goes months (even years, as in the *Family Circle* survey) without sex, he may stray. Even if the man is biologically monogamous (i.e., he does not have the nonmonogamy gene), he can stray sexually during this time. However, if a husband's infidelity during this time is the only reason a woman with a new child wants to divorce him, she might want to think long and hard about this. In addition, she should make sure that both she and her husband seek counseling to better understand their true goals and the meaning of the affair.

2) If either partner has lost their sexual desire, monogamy may be at risk. Statistically speaking, it is most commonly the woman who develops low desire (we will address this again later). It is

important for the person with poor desire to focus on developing enjoyable sexual habits for themselves so that they can understand who they are sexually and work to keep sex as frequent as necessary for the pair-bond to remain monogamous. In America, 15-20% of couples have sex less than once a month. It is a bit hip in the media now to talk about "sexless marriages," but I feel frustrated by people who stop having sex within their marriage and then are devastated when their partner starts getting it elsewhere. I believe marriage is, in part, a commitment to be sexually available to each other. If you have stopped having sex, there is most likely something wrong physically, emotionally or relationally in your life. If the sex is bad, if you are too angry to have sex, if you are too sore or feel too fat or too tired...these are all issues that can and should be navigated with professional help. Meanwhile, let's all agree to be realistic: even though you may both be saying, "it is okay we aren't having sex," and "we will get to it later," if you are 60 years or younger, you are playing with fire. And this fire is one of your own making. When couples have infrequent or no sex, they are at a *very high risk for infidelity or other manifestations of unhappiness* in one or both partners. No amount of denial is going to change this.

3) If marital communication and nonsexual intimacy have dissipated significantly, your monogamous marriage may be in danger. You and your partner might still be having sex, but your general communication and other kinds of intimacy may have become nonexistent, rote, boring or dispassionate. If this goes on for months or years, and if one of you is biologically nonmonogamous, marital infidelity will most likely ensue. A new partner provides what the brain needs—novelty, excitement, communication, intimacy and passion. Decide if you value each other enough to forgive past hurts and to prioritize each other and the playtime needed to fall in love again.

Stay Busy at Home

The most obvious and direct way to keep the home fires burning is to make sure there is lots of good, healthy sex at home. People who go to work or leave for a weekend feeling horny because they haven't had sex recently are much more likely to "encounter" a situation that will lead to infidelity, especially if they drink. Sexually satiated people are far less likely to take note of that second look from the handsome man at the gym or the low cut blouse of their intern.

What is "good, healthy sex at home"? It is important to remember that the *average* number of times fertile, monogamous couples (between 25 and 40) have sex is between two and three times a week. This number is fairly consistent among cultures and has been so across time. It is also an amount that has been shown to *best preserve male erectile function.* Couples who have sex two to three times a week report better sexual satisfaction and overall relationship quality. Although some fertile-age couples have more and some less, having dramatically less sex, such as once a month or even only once a week, can negatively impact sexual function in both partners. It may feel "easier" not to have sex several times a week, particularly if you are zoned into your daily computer time or feel comfortable together watching TV, but honestly it is well worth shutting these off. Electronics may prove to be the ultimate monogamy buster!

As my first marriage came to a close, I began applying to a number of graduate schools to begin my PhD program in reproductive physiology the next fall. During my practice, I had completed an experiment on embryo transfer in cattle, and the data was chosen for presentation at an international veterinary meeting in Ireland where I knew I could also meet some of the professors I was interested in working with. At the conference opening dinner and dance, I met a tall, blonde, blue-eyed German who worked for the World Health Organization. In fact, he had the job I wanted! A genetics conservationist, he traveled around the world collecting sperm and embryos from endangered livestock species in remote regions in order to freeze these cells for future use in diversifying the gene pool in food animal production.

Peter was a "mover and a shaker" and every bit as strong-minded as me. I ended up staying at his hotel the third night of the meeting. We had fun together, and I was ecstatic when intercourse didn't hurt. I was really attracted to him, and I had gone off birth control pills so the "juices" flowed more naturally. Peter enjoyed spending a long time in bed before and after lovemaking, and that was exactly "what the doctor ordered" for me. I remember thinking that maybe, just maybe, some of my previous issues with my sex life were exacerbated by a lack of sleep, time pressures and a glut of stress. I started feeling hopeful that, going forward, sex might become a less complicated aspect of my life.

After a few snuggly nights under thick Irish comforters (they don't heat Irish bedrooms), Peter headed back to Germany, inviting me to visit him in Munich. For my part, I headed out in blustery January weather to southern Ireland, carrying my awkward and huge suitcase (I wasn't an experienced traveler back then). I bumped around small towns on the bus route, hiked to abandoned castles in the middle of pastures and then made the twenty-four hour trip by boat and train to Germany. Being a traveling newbie in Europe, I didn't realize my Irish pounds (currency) wouldn't work on the train, so I had no funds for drinks or food, making the trip stressful and uncomfortable.

Near the end of the trip, I met Marcus. He spoke no English (and my German is elementary), but he did have a few snacks to eat—which made him my immediate friend. Interspersed with laughter, we tried to make conversation through language, drawings, and hand gestures. Once we arrived in Munich at midnight (during a major holiday), I called Peter. His housemate told me he had left town to be with family and would be back the next day. No problem…until I called four or five different hotels, all full. Now I was getting worried. Marcus had stood by to make sure I would be okay and then told me I could crash at his hotel—it had two beds, and he was heading on to Salzburg the next day. I agreed and thanked him. On the way to the hotel, we went out for a beer and dinner. I was exhausted from the 24-hour train ride with little to eat or drink, so we soon left for the hotel where I "passed out" right away on one of the twin beds. I had expected to get some rest and leave early the next day.

Later that night, I woke up on my stomach with Marcus holding me down while he penetrated me from behind with his hand over my mouth. It took me a minute to even register what was happening. Until that moment, I had not ever really realized the difference in size and strength between a man and a woman. He outweighed me by a good seventy-five pounds, and he had the advantage of having me flat on my stomach. Because of, or in spite of, my struggling and trying to bite his hand, the whole episode didn't last long. Afterwards, he rolled over and fell asleep. I got up, threw on the jeans I had taken off earlier, grabbed my suitcase and went to the communal bathroom down the hall where I showered and spent the night sitting on the floor in the corner, unsure what to do. At daybreak, I left the shower and went to the train station where the rhythm of normal life soothed my mind.

When I saw Peter the next day, I mentioned nothing about what had happened. In fact, I never really told anyone about it for years. I felt like if I didn't talk about it, it would cease to exist. And the rape itself—well, I viewed it as just one more in a string of "unfortunate" sexual encounters in my life. It wasn't the first time in my life that sex had been painful. Mostly, I felt incredibly stupid for having put myself in that situation. This was long before cell phones. I hadn't registered at the front desk. In fact, no one in the world knew where I was! In many ways I was grateful that it hadn't been much worse.

I am glad that during those months after Munich, I made the choice of deciding not to see this event as "the end of my life." Years later, I have determined that my instinctive reaction—both to be angry but also to take this in stride and learn from it—was the right choice for me. As I have told my kids, "no matter what you do, it is impossible to fully avoid danger." For me, to live a risk-free, boring life has always been my greatest fear, even when things have not turned out as planned. I will never stop doing the things I love…with someone or even by myself.

I also know that not all sexual abuse situations are the same—some are primary people in one's life, some go on for years and some are very violent. In the end, life continues to happen, and the ability to accept the parts of oneself that have been changed is essential. I often think of a line from the poem "Invictus" which I have memorized. "I am the master of my fate," writes the poet, "I am the captain of my soul." I feel this line as a refrain about many things in life, including sexuality. We are who we are. No matter what happens, we must *never* let anyone take our psychological or sexual self away from us. No matter the battle we have to fight to get to the other side of pain toward pleasure and purpose, we must fight on for ourselves, so that in the end we remain the captain of our sexual self, as well as our soul.

Knowing What To Do When Bad Things Happen

Young people—and younger women in general—are at risk of rape, with 6% of eighth-grade girls in an Oregon survey reporting they had been raped. By the time they are 24, this increases to 11% of

American women, but it can be higher in certain demographics (e.g., military, college students, poor or urban). A large survey of 15,000 people found lifetime attempted "nonvolitional sex" was experienced by 19% of all women and 5% of men. Completed forced sex acts occurred with 10% of the women and 2% of the men. The mean age for the occurrence was 21 years old for women and 19 years old for men. Individuals the victims knew usually perpetrated the attacks, including: current or former partners (41% of women and 23% of men), family members or close friends (20% of women and 30% of men), acquaintances (21% of women and 30% of men) and more rarely a stranger (15% of both women and men). *Fewer than half* of the victims told someone what had happened to them.

I hope you will let your kids know it is always safe to tell you if anything such as this happens, no matter what the circumstances (e.g., no judging the "dumb" things they did to get there). Tell them to demand, clearly and loudly (if possible): "STOP, I do not want to have sex with you!" Encourage them not to worry about hurting anyone's feelings by loudly yelling these words, especially since most rapists are people they know, which can lead the kids to feel an initial reaction of embarrassment.

Most of us don't tell our kids these things because we are afraid that speaking of it will bring it into being. In addition to our girls, boys need to know about this, especially if they are in isolated mentoring situations (such as sports or religious activities) where male-on-male attacks are common. All kids should know to take the following steps if they or a friend are assaulted.

- Get away from the attacker to a safe place as fast as you can.

- Call 911 or the police. Don't worry if you feel unsure about what to call what happened (e.g., was it rape?)—let them help you determine this.

- Call a friend or family member you can trust. You also can call a crisis center or a hotline to talk with a counselor. One hotline is the <u>National Sexual Assault Hotline</u> at 800-656-HOPE (4673).

- Do not wash, comb or clean any part of your body. Do not change clothes, if possible, so the hospital staff can collect evidence. Do not touch or change anything at the scene of the assault.

- Go to your nearest hospital emergency room as soon as possible. You need to be examined, treated for any injuries, screened for possible sexually transmitted infections (STIs) and given pregnancy prevention medications if needed. While at the hospital:

- If you decide you want to file a police report, you or the hospital staff can call the police from the emergency room.

- Ask the hospital staff to connect you with the local rape crisis center. The center staff can help you make choices about reporting the attack and getting help through counseling and support groups.

- Adapted from the Office on Women's Health, *womenshealth.gov.*

———————————

During the next nine months (after I returned to the U.S.), Peter and I had the perfect long-distance relationship, with a bonus: we were always on vacation when we were together! There was nothing real or day-to-day about it. He visited me a few times in the U.S., and I saw him in Germany again. We spoke on the phone once a week. I started imagining a German wedding and little *Kinder* running around the orchard of our dairy farm in Bavaria. In terms of the sex, Peter was a skilled, playful lover in bed, but our sex was pretty vanilla. In the end, I think this was good; it was a healing time, relieving me of much of my fears that I might be some kind of freak in intimacy. By reviewing my past marriage in the light of my relationship with Peter, I realized that while marriage-in-sexual-ignorance-of-one-another fits with much religious doctrine, it can also doom couples to years of sexual frustration and lack of self-realization. Loneliness, infidelity or divorce can be the only options if these couples don't have the tools to communicate through their issues or know how to find help (which is often difficult because of the lack of experience in the couple's background).

Finally, in the end, Peter went to work in Mongolia collecting embryos from yaks, and it was time for me to head to Cornell to start my PhD studies. In actuality, I was also starting what would end up being my life's work, studying the science of sex in all its incredible, cellular detail.

Chapter 7

The Incredible Journey

As I pulled into Cornell University in Ithaca, New York in my old Chevy pickup, I had no job, no husband and no place to live. I did have my beloved Doberman, "Hera," my grandmother's antique rocking chair and a pretty clear idea of what I wanted to study. I had chosen Cornell so that I could work under Dr. Robert H. Foote, one of the pioneers of artificial insemination and in vitro fertilization. Upon my arrival I told Bob that I wanted to use my PhD work to look at how sperm are held in the female's Fallopian tube (FT) prior to fertilization. "What factors from the tube make sperm ready to fertilize the egg?" I wondered. Back in 1987, as I started my program, the FT was primarily viewed as just a pipe for sperm to swim along to encounter the egg. But I had an instinct that something more complex must be going on between the FT cells and sperm that enabled and coordinated fertilization.

I explained to Dr. Foote that I wanted to grow FT cells in a Petri dish so that I could watch how they communicated with sperm to optimize their ability to fertilize the egg. I planned to begin this study using tissues from cattle and horses as research models and then move onto human tissues. Originally, my long-term goal was to use this information to develop a new type of contraceptive targeted specifically at stopping these sperm changes in the FT so that they could no longer fertilize the egg. In a twist of fate, I instead ended up developing a product to optimize sperm function and human fertility!

Sperm 101

In order to better understand my research over the years, we need to review basic sperm physiology. The journey of a single sperm cell from the man's testicles, through his penis to the woman's vagina, to the Fallopian tube and ultimately into the egg to make a new person is (to my mind) the most amazing aspect of human physiology. I used to tell my students, when I taught physiology, that the Fallopian tube is the center of the universe, since it is where we each are conceived and where our individual universes started with a big bang between sperm and egg. Although much more is now known about these events of early reproduction, very little was understood thirty years ago in 1987, especially when it came to the tiny Fallopian tube tucked deep inside the mom's body. To help you better follow my discoveries back then, I will lay out the current understanding of this physiology as it stands today.

Nature stores sperm in the male's scrotum outside of the body cavity at a lower temperature than the rest of his body because heat matters a great deal to sperm health. If a male runs a fever high enough to raise scrotal temperature to his internal body temperature for a day, abnormal or low sperm production for two months or more can result. Thus, sperm (like far more things about males than we tend to realize) are fragile. Their genetic material (the DNA in the chromosomes) is the most easily damaged or broken of *any* cell type in the human body.

This does not mean they are helpless. The male reproductive system makes up for its fragility with quantity—via a constant turnover of fresh sperm. In fact, tens of millions of sperm in *each* ejaculate compete to win the right of fatherhood. No weakness or damage is minor in a sperm cell's DNA. Every single piece of the millions of units that make the baby's genes is critical for a healthy outcome.

Females, for our part, know how fragile sperm are at a physiological and cellular level as our bodies work to keep sperm alive for a week or more (the longest report is twenty five days) as they wait for the egg. The female stores and prepares the sperm for entering the egg at the right time by facilitating "capacitation," a unique series of events that unlock the sperm's outer membranes so they can fuse with the egg.

To imagine how capacitation works, pretend you are in the lab with me: put a sperm and an egg together in a Petri dish. You'll see that no fertilization will occur in this Petri dish unless the scientist adds *external* chemicals to physically change the sperm membranes so they become capable (i.e., capacitated) of fusing with the egg. Only then can the sperm deposit their DNA into the egg. In nature, the Petri dish for sperm capacitation lies inside the female's FT. While resting in the tube attached to the FT cells, the sperm encounter sugar-proteins (we will call them "FT sugars") that act as natural, membrane-unlocking mechanisms for the sperm. Once ovulation has occurred, these FT sugars trigger capacitation, releasing sperm in wave after wave in a coordinated fashion. This mechanism happens because the FT cells are amazingly "smart": they know that once sperm are capacitated, they die very quickly, within about an hour. They also know that this rapid death is a good thing—nature doesn't want degenerating sperm with damaged DNA to hang around and inadvertently fertilize an egg. By constantly releasing a few powerful capacitated sperm at a time, the best sperm are always available even if it takes the egg a bit longer than expected to make its journey down the tube.

For our purposes, let's think of the cells lining the inside of the Fallopian tube as highly-trained flight attendants in the First Class cabin of a long overseas flight. They provide food and drink for the sperm in the FT and tell the sperm when it is safe to remove their seatbelts and move about the cabin (after they are capacitated) so that these capacitated sperm can move up the tube to meet the egg.

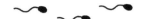

Before I headed to graduate school, my overall career goals had changed away from the animal conservation work. Instead, I had developed an interest in finding safer, better methods of birth control during my PhD. This redirect followed my own negative experiences with birth control pills and my experiences in India. During my time there I had stayed with an upper-class Catholic family who had lost both their daughters (and only children) to illegal, "botched" abortions. Their story affected me deeply. These people could afford the best healthcare available, but their daughters had turned to hidden alleys to avoid embarrassing their family with their sexual lives. One by one they had died. This shocked me. Elsewhere on our trip, I met men and women who had developed crippling, chronic complications following vasectomy surgery or tubal ligation sterilization procedures performed in outdoor tents around the countryside of India. These people were ill or dying trying to prevent unwanted pregnancies. And as I remembered how poorly my body tolerated oral contraceptives, I was convinced (and still am) that science and medicine can do better than the hormonal contraceptives that constantly flood our whole bodies with hormones to fool them into thinking we are pregnant so we won't ovulate (which is how hormones such as the pill, implants or injections work). Stopping sperm cellular changes specific to fertilization of the egg using targeted antibodies or cell chemistry could provide contraception without such side effects.

But that same year I returned to school at Cornell, President Reagan and Congress removed funding for contraceptive research from federal agencies. As I laid out my plan, Bob sighed deeply and said, "It's a great idea, but we can't get it funded via the angle you want. Let's look at it from a different way." I was devastated at first but then saw the wisdom of his thoughts. Under his direction, I switched my research goals from studying the FT environment in order to find safer, targeted contraceptives to studying it to find new ways of combatting *infertility*. I could study what the FT cells were doing with the sperm and how they were doing it as long as I did so in order to help couples become pregnant. This was, of course, an example of serendipity. My new goal was an unexpected detour on my scientific journey, but this course change would eventually lead to development of the world's first fertility lubricant, Pre-Seed. Grateful for these opportunities I have had throughout my life, I will never forget those who live in places where birth control is something to die for.

Female Reproductive Rights

As I work with young women in America today, I see many who take the rights they have for granted. Lack of access to safe abortions isn't real to them. They don't know girls who died from backstreet abortions. They don't have sisters or aunts who are sterile from these procedures. They may understand the image of a coat hanger as a symbol of self-induced abortion, but the image is only a faraway picture of a horror they think they will never experience. And yet... because they are women, they should never easily relinquish control over their personal reproductive decisions. Ask the women in Iran, Iraq or Bosnia. What women view as their "rights" can change in an instant, especially if we don't remain aware and politically engaged.

Birth control access and affordability still matter because 85% of unwanted pregnancies occur in women who are not able to find or afford birth control. When women have unwanted pregnancies, throughout history and still today, many will seek any means possible to terminate these pregnancies. Roughly 13% of maternal deaths worldwide are a sequel to abortions, mostly in places where abortions remain illegal and unsafe (i.e., are done by someone without adequate medical training or in facilities with minimal medical equipment). In the U.S., death from legal abortions occurs at 0.6 deaths per 100,000 women. In Africa, where abortions are illegal and unsafe there are 460 deaths per 100,000 women. Worldwide, post abortion complications occur in an estimated 8 to 9 million women per year, especially in Africa and Latin America where over 95% of the abortions are done in unsafe settings.

An anti-abortion or pro-choice position is not about whether one likes or dislikes abortion—nearly 100% of us are actually on the same side of this debate, hoping for a day when there are no more abortions. But a majority of Americans believe that the Supreme Court decision supporting reproductive choice in Roe vs. Wade should be upheld. In spite of this fact, access to safe abortions is rapidly eroding. Between 2011 and 2013, more than 205 abortion restrictions were enacted. This is more than the 189 bills enacted *during the entire previous decade* (2001 to 2010). In 2000, the Guttmacher Institute counted thirteen abortion "hostile" states (states with four or more restrictions on abortion access), but in 2013 as many as 56% of all U.S. women found themselves living in one of now twenty-seven abortion-hostile states. Abortion restrictions in these states have little or nothing to do with patient safety—they are purely aimed at making it harder for girls and women to find or afford an abortion. So many clinics are now closing that access to a legal medical procedure in America often depends on where we live or how much money we have to get to a clinic. At the time of this writing, the last legal abortion clinic in Mississippi is fighting to stay open. Numerous American women now live over 200 miles from any provider clinic; thus, for a teen without money or a car, the clinic might as well be on the other side of the moon!

Radical Center Ruminations - Nearly 90% of Americans believe birth control is moral...but just what kind is moral? Some people wrongly believe that Plan B contraception is an "abortion." These folks are wrong about their science. Plan B is classified by the FDA as an emergency contraceptive that greatly reduces the chance of pregnancy if taken within seventy-two hours after intercourse. Especially when talking with young people, we must help them realize that Plan B does not terminate an established pregnancy. Instead, it stops pregnancy from occurring.

This is important to teach our youth because when they go into a pharmacy, they may be met by healthcare providers with anti-abortion sentiments who will try to block their access to the medication. In a survey of 1,000 pharmacies around the U.S., 20% of people posing as 17-year-olds were told they could not buy Plan B even though they **legally had the right for access to this product.** Plan B is supposed to be stocked out on shelves in stores (not behind the pharmacist) for purchase by anyone (male or female, young or old) who wants to buy it. Knowingly providing false medical information is grounds for governing board sanctions on pharmacists. If anyone you know has received false advice regarding Plan B contraception, contact your State Board of Pharmacy and let them know. We simply cannot allow people in healthcare professions to provide misleading or erroneous information based on their personal beliefs.

Discovery in the Lab

My work on my PhD thesis involved a mix of work in the barn collecting sperm or eggs from my research cattle, harvesting cow Fallopian tube cells from a local butcher and putting all these cells together in the laboratory to see how they interacted under the microscope. I loved growing the layer of FT cells in the lab and admiring their long slender cilia beating in the Petri dish like waving grass. After bull sperm were then added to these dishes, the sperm would swim in and around the FT cilia, with many sperm eventually stopping and attaching to the tubal cells where they were held tight by the FT cilia wrapping around them (the seatbelts in our plane metaphor). Lastly, I would add the round cow eggs to the dish where they would roll gently about, propelled by the beating FT cilia and the swimming sperm with their strong tails. Most other cells grown by scientists in tissue culture just lie flat in the dish (boring), but not these reproductive cells—they move!

One of the most exciting experiences of my life was my first "big scientific breakthrough." It occurred during an experiment in my second year of research. For months at a time, day by day, and week by week, I had been collecting and growing the FT cells and adding bull sperm and cow eggs, but throughout this process, something was missing: the sperm were not capacitating in the dish (i.e., they were not becoming capable of fertilizing the eggs). Pondering this, I began to realize that the FT cells could not form the machinery needed for sugar production in a flat plastic dish. They needed a 3-D structure that felt like a living Fallopian tube. Our flight attendants on this plane had been transferred to a barge with no food or drink of any kind and no comfy seats for the passengers to buckle into. Even though the flight attendants and passengers (the tubal cells and sperm) were both present, the flight attendants had no way to nurture the passengers and no way to let them know when it was time for them to release their seatbelts and disembark to meet the egg.

To help the FT cells differentiate, I tried various methods of growing the cells so they felt more "at home," including finally placing them on a "matrix" of connective tissue collagen so that they could grow taller and more able to secrete sugars like they do in the female's body. One winter day, I finally began to see the FT on the collagen matrix growing to look more like tubal cells in the female body; specifically, they were forming peaks and valleys that were similar to their natural architecture. After a week of growing the FT cells on the matrix and letting their sugar production crank up, I placed bull sperm and cow eggs together on them. The next night, I drove back to the laboratory at 10:00 pm through the ice and snow of Ithaca, New York for my fertilization check. Not expecting too much, I looked into my microscope…and saw *fertilized cow embryos* in the Fallopian tube system! A colleague beside me, Dr. Kim (a proper, older, post-doc from Korea who spoke very little English but who was always there with me in the laboratory late at night) almost screamed in shock as I started jumping up and down, hugging him and shouting, "We did it! We did it!" When we (I!) calmed down, I showed him the brand new, tiny baby calves (only two cells old) dividing in my laboratory Fallopian tube.

Now, finally, I had created cattle embryos in the laboratory without relying on chemical capacitation of the sperm—just using the natural sugars of the FT cells! I had, in our metaphor, reconstructed my plane so that my flight attendants comfortably nurtured their passengers throughout the journey, releasing them hale and hearty when it was time to meet the egg.

My new discovery was one that would ultimately help prove my hypothesis that the Fallopian tube itself is an active participant in fertilization, not just a meeting place for the sperm and eggs. Over the course of my PhD research, I designed and completed experiments supporting the role of the mare's and the cow's FT in not only welcoming the sperm, but also in protecting the highest quality sperm until the egg came, and then helping to capacitate these sperm for fertilization. My breakthrough moment and the work that followed allowed me to write several successful grants, including the very prestigious Physician Scientist Award from the National Institutes of Health, enabling me to continue using my animal model to look at how sperm are stored in the female prior to fertilization.

Discovery Out of the Lab

Outside of my scientific studies, graduate school was an amazing time for my personal sexual development. I could tell by now that I was a relatively high-testosterone woman, ready to love, experiment and discover greater sexual fulfillment. In my first week at Cornell, at a party for new graduate students, I stood against the wall wondering if I was too old for this whole student party thing when a good looking, dark-haired man walked up to me. He placed his arm against the wall, partially blocking me in. Locking his eyes with mine, he said, "If you are Wilderness, I know who you are." Decades later I still vividly recall the feelings of that moment. I felt "recognized" by this person in a way that made me suddenly believe very strongly in reincarnation (in his eyes I remember having a visual flash of an ancient grove of sycamore trees). The word "Wilderness" resonated with me. I sensed at a cellular level that he meant something cosmic, some past when I myself and he and all other living things were part of a sundrenched grove of tall, intertwined sycamore trees near a flowing river.

His name was Teo. And he was a graduate student from New Mexico where his grandmother was a *curandera* (a Mexican healer). We ended up living together over the next few years. Teo and I read all the Carlos Castaneda books together and shared a language of the "worthy opponent," mystical "seeing" and being a "warrior" in life. Years later, when I read Brian Greene's *The Fabric of the Cosmos*,

I saw in print again what Teo had taught me—how the concepts of current physics had long before been explained by mystic Nagual shamans in the Mexican desert, how filaments of light create and connect us (now explained as string theory) and how two types of energies, the Nagual and the Toltec (now explained as boson and fermion particles), keep us contained and safe.

Besides his spiritual understandings, Teo was also a very sexual man. During our relationship I often teased, "Making love is like a religion to you." He agreed. In his mastery of making sex a matter of "spirit," I felt naïve and provincial at first because I really hadn't developed much creatively in the lovemaking realm. I usually just worked to make sure my and my partner's technique allowed me to have an orgasm and to avoid soreness. I certainly had not ventured into a way of being in which sex was a channel for spiritual connection and expression.

With Teo, regardless of our sexual position, I rarely had pain during intercourse or soreness afterwards. I relaxed, trusted his capability to please me and learned I could have not just one sought after orgasm but multiple ones. The difference in how my body responded to Teo fascinated me. It convinced me that our partners' smells, eyes, tongues, sounds and sexual skills matter to us at a deep biological level. I continued to be protective of my parts "down there" (still, and always, searching for underwear and clothing that wouldn't cause irritation), but now there were other things to think about as well!

Teo involved me in more varied sex play, including blindfolding me and tying me up. We bought soft, stretchy, black velvet cloth to cut into strips to tie each other up and a feather duster to tease with. Over time, Teo taught me the joy of being powerless with a man as he slowly explored my body using his hands and even sex toys and a vibrator. And I did the same for him. This made me feel sensual and powerful, so much so that I realized I had never felt those things in this way before. A feminist and independent woman, as well as a scientist, I had believed that a woman makes herself powerful on her own, alone, without dependence on men. But Teo taught me a lot about partnership and about what it felt like to be truly liberated with a friend and lover. There is a beautiful dependency in it—one that nature intended.

Good Vibrations

Vibrators are becoming a mainstream staple of sex in America. If a woman needs an orgasm *now*...with little work or time investment... electronics are just the thing. In fact, according to the latest research, 50% of women ages 18 to 60 have used one in sexual activities as well as 45% of men. Use is highest in married women. In contrast, only a quarter of single women have used one (this needs to improve!). About half the time, women use their vibrator alone, and the rest of the time they use it during intercourse and foreplay with a partner. Most women who use a vibrator (84%) use their vibrator for direct clitoral stimulation while 64% use the vibrator to penetrate inside the vagina.

Several studies have found that vibrator use is associated with better sexual function among lovers. Women who have used theirs most recently report more positive sexual function with regards to arousal, lubrication and orgasm. Very important to all this is that fact we mentioned earlier: women and men who have good orgasms together feel more overall relationship and sexual satisfaction. Vibrators can be, in this context, a very important tool in extending and expanding the love we feel for one another.

Vibrators are primarily sold as novelty items which means there is little FDA oversight on their quality. However, recently trusted names such as Trojan® have taken vibrators mainstream to the grocery and pharmacy shelf. By bringing their quality assurance on board, along with ease of purchase at local stores, Trojan is giving these sex enhancers a much broader appeal. Many of us are now leaving messages for our spouses suggesting, "Honey, on your way home from work, can you stop at the store and get some milk, bread and a new Trojan® Vibrating Ring?"

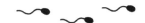

Something Fishy is Going on Down There -- Bacterial Vaginosis

I came to graduate school ready to learn about sexual science in the laboratory, but I also began to realize how ignorant most people are about how to find their own sexual joy. I discovered a yearning in myself to help other people access information so that they could find greater sexual fulfillment. Like me, as I struggled with my sexual dysfunctions, I knew that others often saw flaws in their sexual selves where actually there was beauty, and at worst bore an ignorance of the physiology of their own body which kept sensual self awareness at bay. When issues do occur, many of us lack the knowledge to find the right interventions so that once again we can return to our fully functional sexual identity.

Through one exchange in grad school, I became aware for the first time why the store shelves are weighted down with "feminine hygiene" products to wash, rinse and hide "female" odors. Even with all my pain issues, I had never had problems with "embarrassing" odors. Now I realize, I had been lucky enough not to have ever had bacterial vaginosis (BV). BV is a condition in which women develop the wrong kind of bacteria in their vagina. The most obvious symptom is a strong fishy smell after sex or during a woman's period.

BV impacts over 20 million women in the U.S. Its prevalence is high in some demographics, with 51% of black women having been afflicted at some point. BV is serious. It can cause preterm delivery in pregnant women, and it can increase susceptibility to HIV or other STIs. It can also significantly impede lovemaking because men and women do not like the smell! The smell itself—strong and fishy— occurs from bad bacteria as they are exposed to changes in vaginal pH levels.

The vagina of reproductive-aged women has a low pH of or around four. As women go through menopause, this normal vaginal pH rises to six. But the vagina can also normally and routinely be exposed to a higher pH of seven or eight, including when a woman is ovulating and has fertile cervical mucus; when she is having her period with blood secretions from the uterus; and after intercourse with the presence of semen. Most women will spend about half their days with secretions coming and going in their vagina that seesaw back and forth from the lower pH of the vaginal secretions themselves to the higher pH of fluids coming from their uterus, cervix or their partner's semen. *This is normal physiology.* For women with BV, the contact with these higher pH fluids causes the abnormal bacteria in the vagina to release proteins, making this fishy smell, and impeding sexual enjoyment.

One day a few of my male classmates started talking about how "fishy" pussy smells and why they wouldn't "go down" on women. I tried to explain to these men that women don't walk around smelling like this—that this odor arises when *semen* (with its higher pH) has contacted certain invader vaginal bacteria, which then make proteins that make the smell. "So it's your sperm that's doing this too, okay?" I pressed, "It's not just her. And there is treatment for this from physicians." Frustrating to me was how easily these guys thought that the smell was a normal "female" condition. I pressed on, explaining that women often douched and used other "feminine hygiene" products to cover embarrassing odors without knowing that these strategies can make the BV worse (douching is a strong risk factor for developing BV). The most sobering aspect for me was that these guys were not illiterate people but, rather, graduate students at an Ivy League school in a biological field of study!

A woman's vagina is a very dynamic and resilient organ. It is not a static, passive place with "one" pH. So practically speaking, if you notice a fishy smell from your personal parts, especially after sex or during your period, seek medical help. It isn't normal and it is *not* "you." In the meantime, while waiting for an appointment, a product such as RepHresh® Gel can lower your pH to help speed up the treatment course and combat odors. RepHresh® Pro-B™ Probiotic can also repopulate the vagina with healthy bacteria. Women can also eat a lot of yogurt. Some studies have shown a benefit of applying plain organic yogurt with active cultures (no fruit or junk in it) to the vagina, by soaking a tampon in the yogurt, or by applying it with a syringe to deposit 2-3 milliliters in your vagina. In all cases, check with your doctor to see if he or she approves of any treatment for BV.

Be aware that vaginal disease can also occur when we keep the vagina at too low of a pH. This is called *cytolytic vaginosis*, something many physicians incorrectly diagnose as BV. When this misdiagnosis occurs, you may be instructed to continually use products that lower your natural pH, which will just make the disease worse. If you aren't responding to treatment for BV, try another doctor and ask what other conditions may be present.

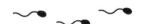

The beauty of an exciting lover can create the illusion of permanence because the sensations seem, at every edge and in every hidden seam, to flirt with infinitude. But in my mind, as I thought about spending my life with Teo, I could sense we weren't long-term partner material. As I began the final stages of my PhD and studied for my theriogenology board exams (in veterinary reproduction), I started to realize that what was magical and mystical about Teo and our relationship wouldn't translate into real life. Neither of us was well enough grounded to be "the adult" when we were together. I don't think I realized it at the time, but at thirty-two years of age, my "biological clock" was ticking. My cells were, quite literally, getting ready for me to become a mom.

Chapter 8

From Maiden To Madonna

During my childhood, I was the oldest of six kids. While my parents worked, I babysat a lot so by the time I was an adult, I didn't see myself as the nurturing type and wasn't really sure I wanted to have kids. In the early 90s, reproduction was something I studied rather than something I "did"... but time and circumstance would change this.

After I graduated from my PhD program in 1990, I began teaching veterinary reproduction at Cornell. I also continued working on my NIH grants looking at the events of reproduction in the Fallopian tube. Back then, most human infertility research looked at problems with women, and there wasn't much funding to look at sperm problems in men. In contrast, in veterinary medicine, a great deal of emphasis is placed on the male, including treatment of male fertility issues. The reason for the animal/human difference is because sperm from many animals have a great deal of financial value, especially if the male is a dog winner from Westminster or a top Thoroughbred racehorse.

I began seeing the gulf between veterinary medicine, in which reproductive decisions are made based on scientific methods to ensure the best chance of successful reproduction, and human medicine, in which politics, culture, religion and greed can impact the treatment of infertility. If a person is infertile, the couple cannot simply replace the husband or wife with a new "better breeding" version. The result is a culture of desperation that makes couples grasp at straws and a medical industry built around expensive, invasive assisted reproduction techniques. These techniques result in over $3 billion in services each year and less than a one in three chance of a "take home" baby for each in vitro cycle. While some people absolutely need assisted reproduction to conceive, it is worth noting that only *0.5% of all babies born in the world (and just 1.5% of U.S. babies) are conceived by assisted reproduction.* That means more than 98 out of 100 children are conceived naturally. In spite of this, a vast majority of our medical research dollars and media attention regarding fertility focus on relatively rare techniques that many people either can't afford or choose not to use, rather than on innovative, practical ways to educate couples and physicians on how to improve natural reproduction.

As I continued my research, I realized that many of the most basic facts of reproductive physiology weren't being communicated to infertile couples and that many physicians weren't even aware of their own knowledge gaps. I saw that my background could help fill in these holes, both for healthcare professionals and the women and men they treated.

At this time, my own mind and heart gradually became more interested in babymaking, and none too soon! Subconsciously, I now realize, I started looking for a father for my future children. Soon after I started working in the clinics at Cornell, I met that father: Hank, a resident in Radiology. He was a smart, capable clinician with deep New England roots. We had a lot in common, from similar family values to a love of the outdoors. He wasn't artistic like Jay, or international like Peter, or mystical like Teo, but he was responsible and solid. Plus, he loved animals, horses and riding. He was perfect for me. We dated for a year before marrying in January of 1992.

Just before we got married, I was offered a new job at Cornell. The university was creating a unique faculty position to work with Congress to draft the first-ever federal guidelines for protecting farm animals used in research. This was to be groundbreaking animal welfare work. At that time, laboratory animals (such as mice and rats) were protected from certain types of studies, but no such laws were in place for domestic livestock. I was excited to play a role in better protecting the sheep, pigs, cattle and horses who gave their lives for science. Of course, I was well-suited for the position because I understood the need for animal research, but I also wasn't afraid to confront investigators who took advantage of the situation and didn't treat their research animals with the comfort and respect they deserved. I planned to start my new and better paying job, with its required travel twice a month to Washington DC, after our wedding.

However, several weeks before our wedding, I had the flu with a fever. Fevers can change ovulation patterns, but I ignored this in all the excitement. Our wedding was a cozy, fun affair at an Adirondack lodge with family and friends, and a decent snowstorm to snuggle up against on our wedding night. Two weeks later I missed my period, and on Valentine's Day I stopped at the grocery store to buy the first pregnancy test of my life. It was positive!

Hank and I sat at our candlelit table wide-eyed and in shock! I remember going in to see my doctor a few days later, still wondering, "How did this happen?" She just laughed at the irony that a PhD in reproductive physiology was stumped by the whole "sperm meets egg" thing. Needless to say we were a bit murky on when conception might have occurred. When it came time for an ultrasound, the doctor measured the baby and looked at her chart and asked, "Would you have had unprotected intercourse around January 16th?" Our wedding night! Of course! That was when I had conceived.

Now, with my pregnancy, I needed to make my first decision with regard to motherhood versus career. Just as my new job was supposed to be starting, with meetings already booked with Congressional staff in DC, I found out I was pregnant. Flying back and forth to Washington from Ithaca several times a month during pregnancy wouldn't work, nor would it work once I had an infant who needed nursing. As so many moms before me, I had to choose between a once-in-a-lifetime job opportunity and motherhood. If motherhood was to be the priority, I needed to decide soon so that I could tell Cornell and slow the growing momentum and planning for interactions with busy national legislators (at least until someone else could be hired).

Wanting to talk my choices through with a trusted confidante, I sought out a talented therapist whom I had known for several years, Mitch Bobrow (author of *Views From the Tightrope: Living Wisely in an Uncertain World*). Catching up with Mitch, I discussed how I felt about this new reality. After listening intently, he said, "From everything you are telling me, eight months from now, you are going to have a baby, and nothing in the world will stop you! Someone else can change the animal welfare laws." I immediately felt a flood of relief and knew he was right! Although the externals weren't "perfect," I really, really wanted this baby, and I wanted the time and space to bond with and intentionally parent my child. From being the oldest of six children, I knew infancy flies past in the blink of an eye, but the bond between the baby and its parents lasts a lifetime. The next day I told everyone involved in my congressional position that I could not take the job.

As my pregnancy advanced, Hank and I prepared to move back West to be closer to my family. I read everything I could find about pregnancy and natural childbirth and found a midwife. As it turned out, even with all my misgivings about *becoming* pregnant, I absolutely loved *being* pregnant. I enjoyed my changing body, found sex during pregnancy exciting and easy, my orgasms were intense and provided a nice break from some of the more uncomfortable aspects of pregnancy. Discovering the wonderful book *Spiritual Midwifery*, by Ina May Gaskin, I followed its instructions for perineal massage and stretching. (Now in its fourth edition, this book is still an amazing resource for natural childbirth). Given my past vulvar pain issues, I wanted to be as relaxed as possible for the birthing pain, and I knew from helping animals give birth that most mammalian females aren't used to the sensation of the stretching vulva as the baby's head starts to crown during delivery. This stretching can make the female tense her muscles and fight the relaxation needed for the birth canal to open so the baby can come out.

Perineal stretching, as described by Gaskin, is an ancient practice involving rubbing oils into the perineum (skin) outside of the vulva and having a partner or yourself stretch and pressure these tissues with fingers so that you learn to breathe through and relax when you feel this discomfort. Every few days you can increase the pressure a bit more in order to both mechanically soften the tissues and teach your muscles to relax when you feel the stretch. It was a valuable practice for me.

I also stayed as physically active as possible during the pregnancy, still doing three to four-hour surgeries on cows up until the last month. On a nice fall day in October, Hank and I went for a five-mile hike (we had actually planned to go two miles but got a bit lost in the forest). The next morning I had fluid leaking out, and I headed into the clinic to see what was going on. The fluid proved to be from torn membranes around the baby; my midwife told me it was time to induce delivery. I remember walking into the hospital, not in labor at all, and hearing other women screaming. I just about ran out of the building. But several hours later I, too, was in labor.

I dealt with this labor and delivery largely by keeping my eyes closed for much of it and imagining being a mare. Horses have the quickest labor of any animal species, averaging about fifteen minutes for Stage 2 labor (the pushing phase) because mares want to get that foal out quickly—lying on the ground is a dangerous place for mom and baby, and the mare instinctively knows to push hard to hurry the process along. With Bob Marley singing, "don't worry 'bout a thing" in the background and my mind intent on mare-like focus, I gave birth to my son, Rayne Dylan. After the birth process was finished, I told my midwife, "That was kind of fun."

"That," she told me, "is something I have not heard before."

My biggest discomfort in the whole process was the involuntary passing of stool during the final pushing part. I was nervous about that beforehand and unhappy it happened during, but hey, you know, shit happens!

Of Breasts and Babies

I approached my new baby with a big heart and also a lot of science. From the moment I brought Rayne home, we made sure he got a lot of time outdoors. His first day home we went for a walk to see all the animals. We knew that now, just like over the past millennia, babies belong outside every day; the parent needs the exercise, and the baby needs the fresh air and stimulation.

We also knew that job number one for me, at least for a while, would be nursing. Everyone reading this book is a mammal—a type of animal that feeds milk to its young. Sex makes babies, mommies make milk and babies are supposed to drink that "homemade" milk. Women did this rather naturally...until the formula industry came along and convinced hospitals to give mommies samples of formula. So now, just when mommy is exhausted and sore from having a baby (and her titties are getting raw from trying to feed the baby, and she is breaking down in tears), daddy and other family or friends will say (trying to be helpful), "It's OK, just give Junior a little bit of formula." But then baby gets full on this, and he won't drink as much milk from mommy during the next feeding which in turn tells mommy's body to make less milk in the following hours. Then at the next nursing time, baby can't get enough milk from mommy, and he is fussy and is given "just a little more" formula again, and pretty soon breastfeeding goes out the window!

There are rare times when moms and babies need that formula, so I am not condemning formula, but when formula becomes the *norm* for feeding our babies, we are straying so far away from Mother Nature's wise intentions that we can expect serious consequences for our children—lifetime chronic illness, food allergies, obesity and many other problems.

With Rayne, I knew I needed to establish milk flow and ease the discomfort of my filling and engorged breasts so I sat in the shower with warm water pouring on my breasts for 15-20 minutes several times a day. This opened up the valves in my nipples and "let my milk down." While a lot of milk washed down the drain, this was fine—the mammalian body produces much more milk than the baby will ever drink, so relieving the pressure this way is not a problem. In fact, milk production in mammals is triggered by what flows *out*. The more milk that flows out of the breasts, the more milk a mom will make. Pressure on the nipple stops milk flow by telling the breast that the nursing system is full and milk production should stop. Given this fact, wearing tight bras or tight clothing when milk is coming in can limit production. And since everything in that first week after Rayne's birth needed to be about increasing milk flow to maximize my production, I sometimes pumped the breast that Rayne wasn't nursing. This kept me comfortable and kept my mammalian system naturally instructing my body to make more milk. Some women will over produce, but most women stop nursing because they feel they don't have enough milk. These tips can help you make plenty of milk—and remember: it is easier to get the system to slow down later than to get it cranked up initially.

Another reason women stop nursing is because the baby never seems to fill up. The first milk that comes out of the breast at a feeding is very watery and is primarily for hydrating the baby. It isn't very filling. As the baby nurses longer, the hind milk from deep in the breast (which has more protein and fat) is taken in by the baby. If your baby is fussy or nurses a long time at a sitting, try nursing out one side in a feeding and then switching sides at the next feeding. This way you make sure the baby is getting the concentrated hind milk in a feeding and not just two sets of watery foremilk (one from each side). And baby will stay full longer from this. This is how I fed both my kids, and it is how calves, puppies and piglets nurse, i.e. from one teat each feeding. You can even pump the side you are not feeding while the baby is nursing. Or use a Milkies Milk-Saver (at *fairhavenhealth.com*), which passively collects this extra milk from the non-nursing side. This product was just selected as one of the best products in the 2014 Creative Child Magazine's Awards.

Your baby desperately needs the nutrients and colostrum (immune system developer) in your milk. Equally important, you both need the bonding. The optimal situation is for you to nurse that baby! Even though there can be many distresses when first nursing—rapid milk let down, chapped nipples and long feeding sessions—if you can get through these first two weeks and stabilize your milk flow, things will get better, and you will be breastfeeding your baby. I encourage you to approach this time like you would Boot Camp or studying for finals. It isn't forever—it just needs your very best efforts. Is it worth it? Yes. Evidenced-based studies (Level 1, our best science) show that children who are fed formula instead of nursing have higher rates of ear infections, diarrhea, sudden infant death syndrome and hospitalization for respiratory tract infections. As these formula-fed children grow, they develop significantly higher rates of asthma,

Type 1 diabetes, acute leukemia and obesity later in life. In fact, each *month* of breastfeeding decreases the chance of childhood obesity by *four percent*. That can really add up!

Studies also show that women who have never breastfed their babies have *three times more* risk of dying from heart attacks or strokes before they reach age sixty-five than women who breastfed at least once in their lives. The decrease in mortality is greatest for women who breastfed for seven to twelve months. Breastfeeding women also have a lower risk of postpartum depression, and they are less likely to develop diabetes or breast or ovarian cancer. For every year of breastfeeding, the chance of developing breast cancer decreases 4%.

Economically, breastfeeding is also advantageous. Women who follow optimal breastfeeding guidelines save between $1,200 and $1,500 in infant formula costs in just the first year. A recent study in *Pediatrics*® estimated that if 90% of U.S. families were to breastfeed exclusively for six months, the U.S. would save *$13 billion annually* in reduced medical costs for babies. Mutual of Omaha reported that healthcare costs for new babies are *three times lower* for babies whose mothers participate in their lactation program and are breastfeeding.

Some women truly can't nurse so, again, I don't point these things out to say your life will be terrible if you don't breastfeed. You must live your life as you need to. But I do want to encourage women to make at least two visits to healthcare providers before they give up on breastfeeding. Women frequently doubt themselves, but your baby will be okay for the time it takes you to call a lactation consultant who will come to your home or to dial a La Leche League Leader. La Leche has a great online forum (*forums.llli.org*) where you can talk to other breastfeeding moms. You can always (24 hours a day) call La Leche League Leaders in your area by finding their numbers online. La Leche League Leaders can help mothers and mothers-to-be with all aspects of breastfeeding. They won't judge you, but they can help you get through that rough first week or two.

If you do choose a formula, make sure you know what is in it. Try to choose one that does not list corn syrup as the number one ingredient (most leading ones do). Also remember that ninety percent of soy and corn in the U.S. is genetically modified. The issue with these foods may be the level of pesticide residue that can be present on the crops.

Best Practices for Breastfeeding

Try these best practices for increasing the chance that you will successfully breastfeed your baby.

- *Avoid* childbirth induction (unless medically needed) and epidural anesthesia. Induction can increase epidural rates. Epidurals increase the cesarean surgical delivery rates and fewer women successfully breastfeed after C-sections. The physical triggers from the baby passing through birth canal are missing after a surgical delivery so that the mom's body makes less milk initially. No one should put their baby at risk by arguing for a vaginal delivery against their doctor's recommendation. But for each step along this pathway fight hard against this continuum of events that lead to higher rates of nonbreastfeeding.

- Manage visitors when you are in the hospital and initially when you return home. Plan and stick to a specific "Visiting Hour" and ask *everyone* to come at this same time. If people straggle in all day, they are likely to impede the most important thing you are doing right now with your baby—breastfeeding. This is *very* important!!! You need time alone with your baby.

- For this first week or two, choose one female family member or friend to mentor you. Having too many opinions can be confusing. She should know how to breastfeed and support you. And she should be willing to go when you want her to leave, without taking offense.

- Don't be afraid to be specific and "needy" in phone calls with your doctor about any issues you are having.

- Call a lactation consultant or a trained woman such as a La Leche League Leader (no cost). Using "lay" people (non-healthcare providers) increases breastfeeding retention by up to *sixty-five percent*. Don't hesitate to call your lactation support people again and again and again if you need to.

- Use a hospital that is "baby-friendly" (shockingly, most aren't certified in this manner—see *babyfriendlyusa.org*) and have your baby stay in the hospital room with you.

- Avoid letting your baby use a pacifier during the first few weeks and instead of placing baby in a separate room, try a bassinette next to your bed for easy nighttime soothing and nursing.

- Get the name and phone number of a local lactation support group before you leave the hospital and *throw out* the formula sample!

Remind yourself every day that the pain and chafing of your nipples is temporary. It is a sacrifice of a few days of discomfort for a lifetime of better immunity for your baby...and better bonding between you two. There is no feeling on earth like that of snuggling skin-to-skin with your child as baby draws in the milk your body is making.

When you do breastfeed in these early days of your child's life, get naked, recline, lie down or find some other way that lets you relax. Let someone else take care of other things and other people. This time will not last forever; you will move to the other side of it faster than you can imagine.

Radical Center Ruminations - The United Arab Emirates recently made breastfeeding of children through age two a legal requirement for women. This does seem extreme; nonetheless, it is likely scientifically and socially justified given the actual healthcare costs and long-term impacts (for both women and infants) of not breastfeeding. Medically, economically and psychologically this law is supported by science. Although two years may be more than our American society can handle, we need to bring our culture into balance with our physiology. Nursing mothers need to be accommodated throughout society by giving them the time and place to feed their children and to pump breast milk for them if they choose. Also, the links between delivery induction, epidurals, C-section and failure to nurse need to be discussed more, and attempts made to replace their use with better medicine.

Sex After Babies

Most of us love having the giant full breasts of a nursing mom, but milk leakage is also part of it. Some men enjoy the taste of breast milk and find it sexy, others don't. Rest assured that after the first month, your milk flow will stabilize, and it will be less common to have milk leaking out during foreplay and intercourse. When I didn't want to deal with it when making love, I found the easiest way to stop milk flow was to use a sports bra. You can find some that look sexy and feminine and if they are low cut, your partner can caress your breasts and enjoy them without the milk. The pressure of the tighter bra on the nipple will help stop flow, and the thicker sweat-absorbent bras will absorb any small amounts of leaked milk.

For an entertaining read and some tips to get things going between new parents, check out *Love in the Time of Colic: The New Parents' Guide to Getting It On Again* written by Ian Kerner and Heidi Raykeil.

Postpartum Depression – Hormones and Genes, NOT Poor Mothering

About 15% of women struggle with postpartum depression (PPD), including feeling an overwhelming sadness and hopelessness after the birth of their child. Many people perceive women with PPD as weak and view it as certain evidence that these women are "bad mothers." Women with PPD often feel on a daily basis that they can barely move or cope with caring for themselves, their new baby or other family members, such as baby's siblings or their own spouse. At a time they "should" be happy, they often live lives of silent desperation as they try to hide their condition for fear that others might see them as flawed or think they don't love their new baby. Luckily, the true causes of PPD are just now coming to light. A recent study found differences in genes (actually 116 differences!) between women who developed PPD and women who did not. Amazingly, they found these differences in the third trimester of pregnancy—meaning that even before the baby was born, they could predict 88% of the time which women would develop PPD. All women in the study had similar blood estrogen levels, but the PPD group was more sensitive to *changes* in estrogen levels after childbirth.

Estrogen normally regulates serotonin, the "happy" chemical in our brain. Estrogen creates serotonin receptors, but it also slows serotonin's natural breakdown in order to ensure an ample serotonin supply to bind to these receptors. In women with PPD, their bodies begin to panic with the declining estrogen, and the ability to regulate normal serotonin levels is thrown into chaos. A woman's love for her baby and her capability as a parent have no bearing whatsoever on whether or not a woman will develop PPD. PPD is caused purely by a chemical reaction as changes in estrogen levels in a woman's body stop serotonin from doing its mood-stabilization job.

Until there is an available blood test for PPD, how can you know if you may be prone to this disorder? Women who have more dramatic mood swings during their premenstrual time or who have female relatives who have had PPD may want to discuss warning signs with their physician. These characteristics suggest a possible genetic sensitivity to changing estrogen levels and an increased risk for PPD. Learn about and discuss with your physician new approaches to treating PPD (such as estrogen patch therapy). Also, part of the confused estrogen signaling in women with PPD is related to increased oxidative stress in these women's bodies. Decreasing oxidative stress by lightly exercising, eating healthy foods and taking vitamins may help the receptors in women's bodies "see" the estrogen in their system better. These simple approaches may sound "canned," but they have a physiologic mechanism in which they can make a difference. Gain support from others and rally internally to walk with your new baby for 15 minutes or more twice a day and to eat that salad rather than ice cream. Try these simple steps one day at a time then journal to track and determine what makes you feel better. Know that you are not the problem, but by getting help and making healthy choices, you can become part of the solution to your postpartum depression.

Our new family moved to the Pacific Northwest in January 1993. Hank and his dad drove the U-Haul across the white, icy roads during a huge snowstorm while Rayne and I flew above it all. After we reunited in Spokane and spent four nights in a motel, we found a small house to rent. With no income, we were both highly motivated to get our new referral veterinary practice up and running. Many days would find Rayne playing in a clean dog cage at the clinic while his Dad and I worked on installing new equipment or on a critical case. In the space of less than a year, I had a new husband, a new baby, a new job and a practice. Things were crazy busy as I learned to balance motherhood and my other roles!

During that first year, our referral veterinary practice in Spokane flourished as we provided board-certified specialty services across Eastern Washington and Idaho. As the only theriogenologist in the region, I was on call 24/7, collecting and shipping semen from champion dogs, horses or even llamas to distant females around the world, or assisting with difficult birthings of valuable offspring. I began to realize that being on-call for clinical practice wasn't going to work with motherhood. Animals breed and birth at odd hours, hours that were not consistent with our parenting schedules. By this time, I also realized I was missing scientific research.

Many questions remained for me about sperm and the Fallopian tube (my mind would often wander to design new experiments while I was giving oxygen to newborn puppies or checking cattle for pregnancy). Eventually, I called my mentor and program director at the National Institutes of Health, Donna Vogel, to see if there was a way to continue my science in the Pacific Northwest. Laboratory research, I knew, would fit better with motherhood because it could be scheduled with part-time hours. After quick hellos with Donna, I told her I was concerned that I may never receive research funding again because of taking time off to parent my son at a stage when my peers (mostly men) were gunning for more money and bigger labs.

"You're in luck," Donna assured me, "We have a program exactly for investigators like you. It is basically a re-entry program to help bring people who are good scientists back into research and to get them going again." This was welcome news! But in order to receive grant funds, she explained, I would need to develop preliminary data. I would need to head back to the laboratory again (and quickly) if I wanted to get in a grant application by the upcoming funding deadline!

Chapter 9

Meanwhile Back At The Fallopian Tube

Hanging up the phone from my call with Donna at the NIH, I knew I had no time to waste if I was going to have preliminary science for my grant in time to make the next funding cycle. Luckily, being a new mom had given me plenty of time to think about what kind of experiments I wanted to do next in my Fallopian tube research. I also knew just who to call for help to complete these necessary studies. Previous to our Spokane relocation, I had contacted Dr. Ray Wright at Washington State University to learn about the science network in the region. Ray is a preeminent embryologist who did initial work to help physicians and scientists categorize the health of embryos. Before Ray's work, the medical community didn't know for certain what a healthy embryo looked like (no one had seen very many of them before). He used cattle embryos as a model to reveal normal developmental markers for embryo growth over time, or what we call "stage for age." These models were then used as the basis for understanding human early embryo growth, including if an embryo was poor quality.

Like many animal embryologists, Ray eventually brought his knowledge of sperm and embryos into human fertility. He and his physician partner helped establish the first in vitro fertilization (IVF) center in Spokane. By the time I met with him, he had worked with infertile human couples in Eastern Washington for years and knew many of the gynecologists in the community. Ray let me know that he could connect me with physicians to find infertile couples for my research. These physicians could also help me enroll patients who would donate their Fallopian tubes to our studies while undergoing hysterectomies.

After figuring these steps out, Ray and I sat back on the counter stools in his fertility lab and talked about the challenges of semen sample collection for men going through fertility testing and treatment when all the lubricants on the market killed sperm. We both knew that the men who were going to provide sperm for my studies needed to masturbate into a container to provide a semen sample, but they could not use any soap, gel, cream or oil to lubricate the process. They couldn't make the process feel slippery and sexy, and a dry hand job is just not as "productive." In fact for about one in five guys, it won't work at all this way. Ray also reminded me that when ejaculation occurs without a lot of excitement for the man (such as when collecting a sample for testing), he produces fewer and lower quality sperm than when he feels highly turned on during ejaculation. We talked about the need for a nonspermicidal lubricant (a "fertility" lubricant) that would help optimize sperm production for these men and could also be used by any couple when lovemaking became "babymaking." Little did I know, chatting with Ray as he measured sperm counts from different patients, that these discussions would be life-changing for both me and for millions of TTC couples in the not too distant future.

Being Excited Matters to Reproductive Success

From both animal and human studies, we know that if the male isn't really excited or turned on when ejaculating (such as during the clinical experience of collection at a doctor's office or in the bedroom of a couple "having to have" sex during the woman's fertile time), he may not make his best sperm. Sperm quality and numbers in the ejaculate can be poor for these guys, *even if he is a totally healthy, fertile man.* Sometimes men are misdiagnosed as having male factor infertility or poor sperm quality just because the collection experience wasn't stimulating enough. No diagnosis of poor sperm quality should ever be made before two samples have been provided and evaluated between two and four weeks apart.

Being able to use a fertility lubricant like Pre-Seed can also result in better sperm samples from some men. Recent clinical studies from independent fertility labs around the world have shown that Pre-Seed *is safe* for sperm collection and can improve the collection experience. This sperm-safe lubrication can now help men produce the best sample possible for testing or treatment of fertility issues. But of course, there was no Pre-Seed in 1994 when I met with Ray.

As I prepared to get back into research, I reviewed all the new science in the area of Fallopian tube function. It was fascinating to see the advances in science that had occurred during my absence from the field. It was also gratifying to learn that my doctoral work had added to our overall understanding of FT and sperm physiology. Specifically, in subfertile animals we had found some abnormalities in these interactions that might also occur in humans and cause infertility. But first we needed to confirm that human sperm-FT interactions were similar to that of the other species studied. Of interest, the Cornell work had shown that older females lose their ability to make the FT sugars that capacitate sperm, so the FT can't promote fertilization as well. Similarly, poor fertility male animals produce sperm that are unable to attach to FT cells and undergo these necessary changes prior to fertilization. If we could prove that human FT had the same protective and nurturing effect on sperm as that found in our animal models, it seemed likely that we could show that disruptions of these events could lead to fertility failure in people as well.

In addition to studying if human sperm were stored with the woman's FT cells while waiting for the egg, like sperm in other species, I also hoped to learn if interactions with FT helped select sperm with the best quality DNA to create the healthiest baby. To prove this, I would need to be able to look inside the sperm at their DNA structure. I would need an expert doing cutting-edge work to visualize the genes inside the sperm (their chromatin). A review of the literature showed the obvious person for this work: Dr. Don Evenson at South Dakota State University.

Dr. Evenson had developed a test to see if sperm DNA was intact or broken called the Sperm Chromatin Structure Assay (SCSA®). His groundbreaking research had shown that sperm DNA damage can cause infertility, pregnancy losses and even disease in offspring (such as childhood cancer). Prior to Don's work, sperm were either considered healthy enough to fertilize an egg or too damaged to take part in fertilization within the woman's reproductive tract. It was not yet understood that sperm could look good to physicians or to the egg but carry bad DNA causing genetic defects in the baby. Also unknown was the concept of screening a man's sperm to see if sperm DNA damage might be the cause of his "infertility." I read Don's critical work and hoped he would collaborate with me on these novel studies to look at FT selection of sperm with high quality genetic material.

The Fragile Seed

Sperm are a package of male genes, each carrying the dad's DNA for the baby, with a whipping tail to deliver this genetic information to the egg. A man's other cells (nonsperm) have a routine mechanism that manages repairs when their DNA becomes broken from exposure to the environment or toxins. In contrast, sperm have no such repair capability even though they need a great deal of protection because DNA damage in sperm can lead to fertilization failure, early embryo death, miscarriages or diseases in the offspring, such as birth defects or childhood cancer. To protect the sperm's DNA during ejaculation, the man's semen has high antioxidant levels. Interestingly, the semen of infertile men only contains half the level of antioxidants (on average) of that seen in the semen of fertile men, showing just how critical these protective factors are for launching healthy sperm through the woman's reproductive tract. Once inside the vagina, the sperm leave the ejaculate and swim through the woman's cervix, where they are at risk again for DNA damage with no seminal antioxidants to protect them. But sperm can make it to the FT within minutes of ejaculation. In designing my experiments, I knew the woman's body must somehow provide the antioxidants for the sperm as they wait in the FT for days (or even a week or more) for the egg to come.

I wanted Dr. Evenson to use his SCSA® test to look at the health of the DNA in sperm that the FT cells had selected as the candidates for fertilizing the egg. I also wanted him to see if this interaction with the FT provided protection for the sperm's DNA over time as they waited for the egg. After mapping out my experiments, I called Dr. Evenson and left a message: "I'm a person you don't know from a lab you've never heard of, but I really appreciate your research and wonder if you would work with me to see if Fallopian tube sugars protect sperm DNA." Though I didn't expect to hear back from this famous man, he did call me back, and within the day! We talked for an hour about my hypothesis and what potential experiments he could help me with. I knew I had found a kindred spirit in science as I hung up.

My "Great" Discovery

With Drs. Wright and Evenson serving as copilots for my grant application, I just needed to complete my preliminary studies. Although I wanted to do this work with human FT cells, they are hard to come by. In order to do these studies, I would have to wait for consenting women to be undergoing hysterectomies during their fertile time so that I would have access to FT cells with the right sugars. To more efficiently complete the studies before the grant's upcoming deadline, I decided to look for a naturally occurring sugar from another source that sperm could attach to. My goal was to measure sperm DNA quality before and after attachment to a film of this sugar in a Petri dish, similar to what I expected to do with FT cells. This way we could show the feasibility of using Don's SCSA to measure sperm DNA quality for sperm both free in solution and attached to FT cells. As I talked to colleagues about natural sugar candidates for the work, another reproductive physiologist at Washington State University told me about arabinogalactan (AG). This plant sugar is found in high concentrations in the tamarack tree. It protects the trees from cold and disease and was beginning to be used in cosmetics at the time because of its antioxidant properties. As I read about the structure of AG, I could see that it sounded similar to FT-produced sugars that played a role in sperm attachment. If sperm could attach to AG as they did to the sugars in the FT, I could use AG as a model to prove: 1) attachment to sugars helps select the sperm with better DNA quality and 2) that Don's system could be used to measure this selection process.

To see if AG could be used this way, I coated the bottom of a Petri dish with a thick gel of the sugar and then let it dry until if formed a "fruit leather" looking disc. Next I brought in a sample of human sperm, mixed it with an isotonic salt solution and layered it on top of the AG in the Petri dish. In an instant, the AG film dissolved into the sperm solution!

"Ugh!" I thought. The AG was *highly* soluble. The system was not going to work for what I wanted as no sperm could attach to a sugar film that had disappeared. Disappointed, I put the Petri dishes back into the incubator to continue watching the sperm and AG for a day or two more (because even when things "fail," a good scientist always completes the experimental plan). Although I would come back to check on the sperm in the AG over the next few days, I expected nothing more from the experiment—just an average dish of sperm swimming around in an average dish of media… something I had done a thousand times before.

When I returned to the lab the next day, sure enough, the human sperm were still swimming all over the dish in the AG. Under the microscope they looked like millions of tadpoles buzzing around happily—and very normally. After recording my findings for the day in my lab notebook, I packed up Rayne and took him on a hike near our house in the fall sunshine.

The following day, the sperm in both the AG treatment and in the control media (no AG) were still doing as well as expected. But when I compared the percentage of sperm that were motile (swimming) and their swimming speed, I could see that some of the sperm in the control dishes were starting to slow down and circle, instead of moving in a straight line like the AG-treated sperm. Without running any math yet, I could see that the AG-treated sperm appeared somewhat healthier. "Hmmmm," I thought, as I carried the Petri dishes with their sperm back to the stainless steel incubator and locked them back inside.

The next day when I pulled out the Petri dishes and looked at them under the microscope, I started to feel a growing excitement. In a normal, balanced salt solution, many of the sperm would be starting to slow down or die by now, as was true for my sperm in control media without AG. But *with* the AG, many, in fact, most of the sperm were content, happy and dare I say, "feeling nurtured"—as they zipped around.

"Wow!" I thought, and then muttered in very scientific terms, "This is *so* cool!"

As much as I wanted to keep watching the swimming dance of the AG-treated sperm, I verified my measurements and then immediately returned both dishes to the safety of the incubator, avoiding damage to the sperm and inconsistencies to my findings. While repeating my closing ritual and packing up, I didn't dare to hope, thinking instead, "Okay, well, tomorrow they'll be mostly dead."

The next day when I entered the windowless, tissue culture room with notebook in hand, I was a little nervous and excited to see what I would find. I took the AG-treated sperm out of the incubator and put them under the microscope. I turned the dial on the microscope to focus the lens, looked down and saw blurry movement. This was impossible! Then I twisted the dial, hit the focal plane...and clearly saw hundreds of sperm still happily swimming.

This is one of the most unforgettable moments of my life. I had made what for me was an *incredible* scientific discovery. Sitting back in my wheeled office chair in shock, I saw that the AG had protected the sperm, helping them to remain strong, vital and ready to fertilize an egg. At Cornell I had helped discover that Fallopian tube sugars protect sperm and make them capacitate for fertilization, but now, here, it appeared that a natural, similar sugar (one from outside the FT) could also protect sperm. This was the kind of breathtaking finding every scientist dreams of achieving once in a lifetime. I couldn't wait to tell my colleagues!

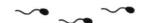

Although as an andrologist I reveled in this earth-shattering finding of AG's protective effect on sperm, I still had an approaching deadline for the NIH grant (which, if awarded, would also pay me a salary!). So, alas, I set aside my racing thoughts of how AG could help human fertility.

Back in the lab, with Ray and Don's help I grew the human FT cells we collected surgically from women and measured sperm DNA quality after attachment in a few samples...just in time to finish the grant. I could now put together the several hundred pages of what would become my First Independent Research Support and Transition (FIRST) award.

Like everyone else applying for this grant, I knew that the 200-page proposal could be perfect (in my eyes) but that it held a less than 15% chance of being funded. Luckily for me, several months later, I got a call from Donna at NIH. She told me that our team had received a fantastic score during the grant review! The panel loved the team we had assembled, the novel proposed studies, the basic science and the transfer of research techniques learned in animal models to human fertility medicine. They were going to award this prestigious grant to my new laboratory!

During the completion and submission of the grant application, my life was a constant balancing act. We had a nanny who came in 12 hours a week to help watch Rayne, but the rest of the time Hank and I juggled our work time. Hank was busy building his veterinary practice during long days. I would work on the computer at home but mostly at night or on the weekends when Hank was able to interact with Rayne and catch up on laundry and dishes. We struggled also to make "grown-up" time for ourselves, including time for intimacy and getting together with new friends in Spokane.

As I continued to learn about AG, I contacted a patent lawyer, Dr. Richard Sharkey, at Seed Intellectual Property Law Group in Seattle. Richard was to become a mighty ally and mentor over the next twenty years. In our first phone introduction, I had to work to keep up with this brilliant man. He had a master's degree in science, as well as his doctorate in law. Richard loves to explain everything in great detail and over the years has taught me the "whys and hows" of patents. But I will never forget my first conference call with him on our old phone anchored to the wall by a cord. Richard booked an hour to walk me through the basics of patent submission. Rayne, at two years of age, was home with me that day. At first he was content to play with toys or the dog. But after about 15 minutes, he became fussy. I grabbed a giant Costco® Cheerios® box and handed it to him on our dining room floor. He nibbled for a few minutes on the cereal but then had a much better idea. He dumped the entire box on the old hardwood floor, happily smashing the pile to bits and rolling in them for the next forty-five minutes while I furiously scribbled notes on my conference call. I was never so happy to clean up a mess than after getting through this critical call without any toddler meltdowns.

Over the next few months, I decided that AG's potential impact on reproductive medicine was profound enough not only to patent but also to warrant forming a new biotechnology company. I invited my colleague who had suggested using AG in the first place to join me in starting the company. We named the company Advanced Reproduction Technologies (ART). Believing that AG could be a game-changer for enhancing human fertility, ART was launched in a sunlit office off the garage of our small home in Spokane. As I sat down to map out the types of products that AG could be beneficially used in, I immediately thought of my conversations with Ray. First on the list of potential products to develop...a "fertility" lubricant that was safe to use when couples were trying to conceive. But that would have to come after grocery shopping, paying bills, making dinner, and getting Rayne to Gymboree® of course!

Modern Parenting - When Work is More Fun

As I worked to balance forming our new company and doing my academic job with the NIH grant, I was also trying to maintain a healthy home for my son. I knew that my parenting journey was simply a variation of the journey that every human parent has lived since the beginning of time: how do I feed, protect and nurture a child while also caring for myself and significant others. Ever the scientist, I studied my situation as a human female and mother as I lived it. I read hundreds of lay and medical articles and books on feeding, schooling, protecting and caring for a new child, as well as on balancing parenthood and work.

Among the books I read was Arlie Hochschild's *The Second Shift* which revealed the intense power struggles that can arise between working couples as they try to balance work, household chores and childcare. One sad finding of her studies in the American workplace was that men and women were actually choosing *not* to take advantage of family-friendly work strategies (e.g., leaves of absence, flex time and working from home). This choice was being made because home life with two working parents was so stressful that parents were seeking escape from the charged home environment by working *more hours than required*. In short, many people simply did *not* want to deal with the hassles of daily home life, sex, relationships and parenting.

Hank and I discussed this book in detail. I felt as a feminist, that many women were missing the boat. We had taken the 1950s model of the distant, overworked dad and created a second distant, overworked parent (mom). Rather than returning to our natural roots of human childrearing—that of a large network of blood and nonblood extended family and community within which parenting flowed throughout daily human work and survival. Our children today had often become a separate "*thing*" to manage a few hours each night. In contrast, for our ancestors, children were part of the process of life as family members wove rugs, collected firewood or herded cattle to new pastures. As career oriented as we were, I knew we needed to have very specific rules for how we would parent or both of us could easily become "lost" in our work.

So we gave the TV to Goodwill, turned on the phone answering machine in the evenings (not listening to the messages until the next day), promised each other we would use no more than twenty hours per week of external childcare and became very selective about who we had time to socialize with. There were only 24 hours in each day, and we needed to use them *intentionally* or our primary goals in parenting wouldn't be met.

The ideals behind our approach were correct, but in the end we forgot to add something to the equation: time for the two of us as parents to maintain our intimate bond. This absence would manifest its effects in our marriage in the years to come. But my goal then and now as a new mom was to find the most natural, healthy way for us to parent our son.

Raising Children "Naturally"

What I learned through my research then, and later, about how parents have cared for human babies over the eons surprised even me with my anthropology minor. The current concept of one dad, one mom and their babies was not how ancient men and women— the providers of our cells and DNA—functioned as "family." Just as our culture treats monogamous pair-bonding as a natural state for humans (in spite of the fact that 89% of all recorded human societies have not been monogamous), we tend to think that the nuclear family is also "natural." But it is *not* natural *if* it operates in isolation. Although the widespread rise of monogamy (one female restricted to mating with one male) was likely a healthy catalyst for some parts of our modern civilization, it still is not the "norm" or a natural state for humans at a cellular level. Similarly, the single-pair (monogamous couple) model of a nuclear family is not a natural human social structure. It places a great deal of stress on parents— and, in fact, parents are running away from the model in droves, making choices that outsource the difficult tasks of child rearing to "KinderCare®" employees they don't even know.

Let's understand our basic biology better for a moment so that we can together envision healthier methods for partnering and raising families in conjunction with the choices we make in mating and marriage. Our patterns of family bonding have existed over hundreds of thousands of years. Throughout that time, the male and female pair-bonding focused on mating and production of offspring, but the joint rearing of offspring did not primarily occur between these same two people. In other words, there were no happy nuclear cave families. How do we know? From a vast library of research in combined sciences—anthropology, biology, ethology, zoology and even from historical texts, such as the Bible. Through many disciplines, we have been able to trace the past of our human DNA to understand how human families have functioned throughout history. The dominant male, who was best suited to father children, was not the kind of guy most of us would want to raise our kids. In fact, caring for human babies wasn't a job for any **one** or even two people in isolation of their larger family or group. Instead, the caregiving *"tribe"* consisted of women and children and the coalitional males who helped support the human social structure by mentoring adolescent males, finding resources and providing protection.

The rise of monogamy and the nuclear family has fundamentally shifted our social structures and the role of men. Men are no longer supposed to spend as much time competing for the right to mate with females—rather they are supposed to cooperate more in the raising of their children. But these relatively "new" roles for both men and women sometimes lead to confusion. Women want men to play an equal role at home, but in many cases women are conflicted about giving up their natural "seniority" as the primary caregiver during the child's early years (our biology is still ancient and drives us to take the lead in parenting our younger kids). In general, many males are dangerously left out of engaging in healthy child rearing in our society, in part because of our emphasis on the nuclear family. Without realizing it, we have nearly destroyed most male kinship systems so that men are now unable to bond with other men in the ways that facilitate broad and effective nurturing of their young.

We have also sadly removed for our sons an important developmental phase, the Right of Passage. This phase was important as it allowed boys to bond with and learn from *mature* men. Sadly, remnants of these systems instead play out for many youth through participation in dangerous gangs. Luckily for some young men (such as my son), people like Tim Corcoran at Twin Eagles (*twineagles. org*) are speaking out more clearly about the need for healthy male bonding and passage rituals. A good resource for understanding how to best raise healthy young men who can be the excellent fathers of tomorrow is Michael Gurian's book *The Purpose of Boys*. Jed Diamond's book, *Stress Relief for Men*, can also help our guys understand their unique biologic needs for intimacy and emotional health. It offers practical advice to integrate attachment based love, the tension releasing use of earthing and the self awareness of energy medicine in a wholly masculine, health creating way.

Although we are at an exciting time in our cultural evolution with regard to individual self-realization, at no other time in human history have we asked one man and one woman to be everything for each other and their children. Science shows us that we need male-centric and female-centric tribes of people around us to love us, and our kids, as we learn how to parent. While our young can benefit immensely from stable, sustained, nuclear units, they are not an inherent or instinctual social system for raising our children, as anthropology, history and our current reality show. Given our cultural evolution away from monogamous marriage, we need to be realistic and invent new ways to provide social stability for kids through a network of elders and other *consistent* adults who remain engaged with our children *throughout* their lives. This isn't a job necessarily for daycare workers, teachers or coaches who come and go in kids' lives. We need to rediscover accountability of local community through extended family and neighborhood. Acknowledging the many wasted social resources and wisdom of our elders should be a first step in this journey.

Hidden Human Interactions

Overall, I hope the science I am sharing helps you look at human sexuality and relationships through the lens of anthropology and evolutionary biology and not just through our transitory culture. Modern life is in part a mask over our ancestral and natural senses. We love, marry, raise children, divorce and feel the full range of human emotions from profound joy to heartrending guilt without fully understanding its source. We live in the veneer of modern life, pretending that several thousand years of religion and a few hundred years of industry and technology are the totality of who we are as humans. But we are much more instinctual creatures than we want to acknowledge and thus are more reactive to an internal language of cues in our relationships. Specifically we all manage our partnerships and families in a world of subconscious interactions between men and women (*intersexual*) and between people of our own gender (*intrasexual*) more than any of us could ever consciously imagine.

An example of intersexual interactions includes the selection process women go through in changing attraction to different men throughout their fertility cycle as we discussed previously. But women aren't the only ones who respond to the opposite sex based on hormonal changes. In studies of customers in strip clubs, men, without ever realizing it, respond to the changing smells and body shape (fuller breasts and hips) of fertile women by offering ovulating lap dancers significantly higher tips (an extra $20 per night) than dancers who are in the nonfertile phase of their cycle. This is an example of instinctual intersexual cues.

In a show of intrasexual cues, socially knit groups of women are more likely to shun a new woman who has high testosterone levels, even before interacting with the woman. Instinctually, via pheromones and smell, these women in their female kinship system sense the high sex steroids in these new women (without having to measure any blood levels) and shun them because the high testosterone women represent a risk to the female social structure. The higher testosterone woman is often more independent and more likely to aggressively seek out the high-genetic-value, dominant males. This woman generally has a higher sex drive and thus is more likely to pursue men who to the other women are already of interest as procreators or nurturers. This new, high testosterone woman threatens other women in competition for the best men. Not surprisingly, these high testosterone women have been shown to be more aggressive and successful in the workplace (but they can also be the woman who is called "a bitch").

Social shunning of these types of gals by other women is a subconscious effort from the majority of women to keep their world safe from the "Jezebels" who would take their men and their resources. That said, these social-outlier women with their high hormone levels are also loners who in the past had to be inventive to survive. They were the women who first made fire or crafted a sling to carry a baby across their backs (think Ayla in the Earth's Children® book series). Their inventiveness and female aggressiveness both challenged and was of benefit to human survival and thriving.

Radical Center Ruminations - About 10,000 years ago, human culture evolved toward the advent of marriage systems to control human mating. In some ways this was a good thing: competition among males for access to breeding females was reduced as family, church and tribal leaders (kinship systems) began prescribing who should marry whom and when (e.g., arranged marriages). As humans settled down to farm, the social stabilizing effect of marriage cut back on violent battles for mating. And as these communities formed, social classes developed in which certain groups of people were able to dictate mating alliances. The new economy and class formations resulted in large differences in wealth accumulation, including access to women.

Occurring concurrently, the rise of agriculture and new marriage rules also cocreated (along with many other economic elements) a marked population increase in humans. As a result, pair-bonding rules became even stricter, and human sexuality became a suspicious activity (a sin). Over time, it also became sinful in society's eyes (especially in highly Puritanical cultures as in the U.S.) to be nonmonogamous.

The rise of monogamy is absolutely correlated with the cultural evolution of democratic societies and women's rights movements: systems that are best for individuals. But species-wide, monogamy may be having some very negative consequences for humans. Researchers have found that of the millions of variations and mutations to our genetic code (DNA) most are evolutionarily very young. As many as 86 percent of the variants that look like they may be harmful to humans have shown up in the last 10,000 years. In other words, just because we are doing something "new" does not mean it is always best. Even more telling, most of these bad genes have only existed for the past 1,000 years. Our "innovations" around sexuality (primarily the advent of monogamy) in the last few centuries may not be necessarily beneficial.

While researchers primarily attribute the rise of "bad genes" to the extreme population boom in humans during the past 10,000 years, I believe concurrent changes to human mating strategies could also be impacting who we are today. During the same space of time that these bad genes have cropped up, natural human mating strategies have been overridden by cultural mate selection (through assigned marriage or love). Now we mate with and marry the one person we fall in love with. While I want for my children this joy and freedom in choosing mates, perhaps we need to find genetic testing for couples that could be used to understand and possibly mitigate any ill effects from our "overrides" of healthy human sexual selection and instinctual mating strategies.

I hope we all come to realize how important it is that we better study and honor our natural DNA foundation as we form partnerships and families. Stopping to understand why we react to other men and women and our partners the way we do can help us choose which of these reactions benefit our long-term goals and which limit our potential and happiness. Parents, use the intersexual cues of exciting pheromones during a wife's fertile time to schedule Gourmet Sex and some fantasy play while the kids stay at Grandma's. Ladies, it may be worth overcoming your negative intrasexual response to your new female boss and choosing instead to learn from her assertive, capable skill set and superior life/work balance.

Chapter 10

A Good Lubricant Can Change The World

In order to complete the NIH grant looking at human sperm and Fallopian tube cell interactions, I needed to find fertile sperm donors. These men would need to have normal sperm counts and quality and have fathered children in the last two years. I decided to start looking for my donors close to home.

Since our move to Spokane, Hank and I had developed friendships with other local families with young kids. We did Gymboree classes together, went to Public Radio kids' concerts or just got together for meals. Much of the topic of discussion and laughter with our friends was sex as parents or, at times, lack of sex as parents. Many of these couples were on round two of babies, so the men fit the benchmarks for my study, and several of them enrolled as donors. These guys were paid $100 for each sample. This created a male "kinship" system of lawyers, doctors and businessmen in Spokane who would pass one another on the downtown streets with a high five while pointing to their shirt pockets. Tucked away inside would be a protected baggie with a semen sample ready for drop-off at my lab. "Getting my new fishing pole with this one!" or "Saving up for Hawaii this month!" they would inform their fellow donors as they saw each other on the street.

Their sample collection stories added a new source of laughter at our parent get-togethers. Our favorites were the guys trying to collect samples before going to work with youngsters banging on the bathroom door—"Daddy, Daddy, open up! Can I come in?"

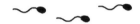

At our house Rayne was nearing three, and Hank and I were ready for another child. I had studied fertility in various species for more than a decade now, but never for a moment did I think my education would need to be applied to me. Hank and I agreed we would stop using the pregnancy avoidance part of the Fertility Awareness Method (my usual birth control), and I thought, "Okay, I'm ready to get pregnant."

What is the Fertility Awareness Method?

The Fertility Awareness Method (FAM) allows a woman to determine the fertile and infertile phases of her monthly cycle. FAM can be used to avoid pregnancy or to achieve pregnancy. FAM is *not* the same thing as Natural Family Planning or the Rhythm Method. It is a very specific monitoring of three physiologic changes in the woman's body that occur when she is fertile:

- her basal body temperature (measured with a special thermometer);

- her cervical mucus quality and quantity (as noted by the woman); and

- her cervical position and shape (as felt by the woman with her finger).

Women who carefully follow the FAM for pregnancy avoidance only have a 5% failure rate (i.e., unwanted pregnancy), which is similar to condoms. FAM is also extremely effective for trying to conceive. Several studies have shown that the highest conception rates are found in women who know how to identify their peak fertility days based on these cervical mucus and temperature changes. To learn more about FAM, read Toni Weschler's book *Taking Charge of Your Fertility* (affectionately known as TCOYF by her fans). Toni also teaches teens this body awareness for their overall reproductive health in *Cycle Savvy*.

After deciding I was ready to be pregnant again, several months passed with no conception. We were now joining the ranks of couples who needed to do something more than just "not trying to not get pregnant." It was time to get serious about using the FAM to optimize my fertility. Through this it became a little too personally apparent to me how having to have sex around ovulation changed the dynamics of intimacy, just as I had heard from so many other couples. When lovemaking becomes "babymaking," sex can feel more like a chore than a deep bonding activity. During this time, I read numerous studies about the impact of infertility on the human pair-bond. I read how couples that continue to find intercourse *enjoyable* during the woman's fertile time are more likely to stay together. In contrast, researchers found that when lovemaking became an added stress for trying-to-conceive (TTC) couples, too many episodes of bad sex could erode the couple's love, resulting in higher divorce rates. I realized that developing a fertility lubricant wasn't just about helping people become pregnant but, perhaps even more importantly, was about helping them *remain in love* and married to their partner.

Sadly, Sally was one such woman I worked with. She and her husband had recently split up after three years of trying for a child. The search for fertility (at least in part) had killed their marriage.

When I saw her for the last time, she told me they had agreed to meet the next day as she was taking hormones to induce formation of an egg. They had agreed that if Sally didn't conceive this month, they would go their separate ways. She needed an injection in her thigh (one that her doctor had provided) to make her ovulate and asked me if I would give it to her. Normally her husband had been around to do this step, but he was driving in from out of town for their rendezvous. It was heartbreaking to see this competent, professional, 37-year-old woman's brokenness as she lowered her jeans and leaned over the back of a chair so I could help her do the only thing she thought could "fix" her world. Sadly, she did not conceive and never would; yet she inspired me to work even harder to push forward a fertility lubricant—one that would give women like her the best chance of conceiving while, at the same time, would help couples maintain the bond of sexual intimacy and pleasure when TTC.

While I was gaining a deeper understanding of the need to fast-track development of a "fertility-friendly" lubricant that didn't harm sperm *and* that helped keep sex fun for TTC couples, my sperm donors on the NIH grant were also reminding me that men needed this lubricant to improve sperm collection for fertility medical procedures. These men were grumbling a lot about how awful dry-hand masturbation was for collecting their samples. Luckily, they forged on in their civic duty to produce these samples needed for our studies and were just starting to yield some fascinating data.

Sperm Live How Long?!

As the work continued on the NIH project, our lab found that human sperm from our donors lived much longer in contact with the FT cells than was currently being taught in reproductive medicine. In fact, in culture with the FT cells, these sperm were living up to 9 days! This was nearly twice as long as what was thought to happen in women's bodies (i.e., 4 to 5 days). We knew from animal studies that sperm from a species do not live *longer* in the Petri dish FT culture system than they do in the real Fallopian tube of the female. Therefore, our data was suggesting that normal sperm survival in women was much longer than was widely assumed. It began to make more sense how women throughout history could have become pregnant from unprotected intercourse just before or during their period (menses). In the past, when women have reported such occurrences, scientists and doctors have challenged the validity of these women's reports, thinking women weren't being honest about when sex occurred. This lack of understanding could have very negative circumstances if, say, a woman had sex with her husband for the last time just before her period. His sperm could then have swum up to attach to her FT cells and rested contentedly in her tubes for several weeks until her next ovulation which would occur several weeks after her period. If a pregnancy resulted from these long-lived sperm, the man might be told that the baby couldn't possibly be his.

Our findings of the varying lengths of time that sperm from different men lived in our FT cell system suggested that instead of supposed infidelity causing the pregnancy in such cases, this man and woman were more likely the reproductive rock stars of our species. The man would have had super-charged sperm that were able to live in the woman's nurturing FT for much longer than the average man's sperm. (The longest report for sperm living in the human FT is actually 25 days.) In addition, this woman's FT cells likely provided a private, executive-class flight environment for his sperm, protecting them in her tubes for weeks longer than biology texts tell us is possible. When the egg was finally ready, these high quality sperm were then released and capacitated to fertilize the egg—all from a single act of coitus occurring up to three weeks earlier.

On the opposite side of the fertility spectrum, I began to introduce sperm from infertile men to the FT system in order to evaluate how sperm from these men interacted with FT cells. We found that these sperm were very limited in their ability to attach to the FT cells and that they did not live as long in their presence as did sperm from fertile men. In fact, sperm from some men *never* attached to the tubal cells and only survived *a few hours* in the system. Sperm from these men looked completely normal under the microscope, but there was something wrong with them. The flight crew on our Fallopian tube jet was kicking these sperm off the plane prior to take off. No nurturing, no pampering—just the boot!

Using Don's SCSA to look at sperm DNA quality, we eventually found that the sperm that are selected for attachment to the FT cells are those with the highest rates of healthy DNA. In contrast, the sperm that are unable or are not allowed to attach to the FT cells are the sperm with more *damaged* DNA. These sperm are destined to be washed out of the tube and destroyed by the woman's white blood cells. Somehow the Fallopian tube cells have an internal mechanism for sensing sperm with "bad" DNA and facilitating their removal from the woman's reproductive tract, even when the shape, the membranes and the tail all look normal in the laboratory. Our studies suggest that the mom's Fallopian tube not only protects sperm during their journey to the egg but also helps select the best sperm to meet up with the egg and make a healthy baby.

The more scientists have learned about reproduction, the more we realize that at the cellular and genetic level, reproduction is a team effort between the woman and the man. When it works, it is because both partners' gametes and physiology have functioned properly. And in spite of centuries of "barren" women being the "cause" of a couple's childlessness, we now know that it takes two to tango. Without healthy sperm, a couple's fertility is compromised.

Ladies, It Isn't Just You

Although infertility is due to a male factor (fully or partially) in at least 40% of infertile couples, there is little support for men going through this challenge. Infertile men are at an increased risk of developing sexual dysfunction, including decreased libido, increased erectile dysfunction and difficulty ejaculating. But babies can't be made naturally without a dad who can get the job done. Men who are experiencing the double whammy of poor quality sperm production and sexual dysfunction need to be seen by a fertility urologist or an andrologist, sooner not later. Specialists in male reproduction have the best training to help men navigate the complex issues around male factor infertility.

For example, Dan and Faith, two friends in our parent group, had been trying to conceive kid number two for three years. Dan had been found to have a low sperm count several months before. Now the marathons of daily sex during Faith's fertile time coupled with Dan's diagnosis were resulting in dramatic sexual dysfunction for them both. They asked me if I could meet them at their house one afternoon to talk about it. Faith explained to me that to increase their chance of success she had begun lying with her hips propped up on a pillow in the assumed "best" position for conceiving during babymaking sex. This made intercourse feel mechanical and unsexy and inhibited Faith's natural lubrication and her ability to orgasm. Not only was this kind of sex disheartening and uncomfortable for Faith, but her obvious lack of enjoyment made Dan feel turned off too. Even though he was able to have and maintain an erection, Dan told me he would start to feel "numb" during this sex and increasingly was unable to "finish" (he couldn't ejaculate). "It is so weird when this happens," he said, looking at the ground.

"You can imagine how this makes me feel," said Faith angrily, "when he can't even get his rocks off to help make a baby." She was referring to the fact that several times lately during her fertile time Dan had not been able to ejaculate at all during vaginal sex, so no sperm ever made it into the vagina! Dan agreed with Faith, "I have never even heard of guys not being able to orgasm. I am worried maybe something is wrong with me. But I am not sure I could even discuss this with a doctor."

As I responded to what they said, I suggested, "Faith, imagine if the only way you could have a baby was if you had to have an orgasm each and every time you had sex." I gave her a moment and then said, "This is the pressure Dan is feeling." I paused, "Dan's role is essential, but he isn't a tool or a machine; he is a human being."

Turning to Dan, I gave him my "jacking up sperm production" talk. Specifically, I suggested the following for Dan as I do for other men with male factor infertility.

1) Order a Sperm Chromatin Structure Assay kit from Dr. Evenson's lab to find out what percent of dad's sperm have healthy DNA. This is an important baseline because infections, work exposure, stress, weight gain, partying and even antidepressants can all make for higher levels of sperm DNA damage. By knowing this baseline, men (and their doctors) can monitor sperm DNA quality over time and determine if lifestyle and medical changes are improving sperm quality.

2) Start taking a fertility vitamin/mineral supplement such as FertilAid™. Our group completed a clinical study for the makers of this supplement and found improved numbers of motile sperm in some men (especially those that smoke). There is currently debate among physicians about supplements for infertile men. But I think *most* men with low sperm counts should try quality

supplements for three months and then redo a sperm analysis, including the SCSA, to see quantitatively if the supplements are helping them or not. And don't take more than the manufacturer recommends (this can actually damage sperm).

3) Ejaculate as much as possible, including masturbating at times, all month long. Men cannot "save up" sperm. In fact, more ejaculation (even daily) actually increases testosterone levels as well as sperm production and quality.

For both Dan and Faith as a couple, I suggested a new approach to babymaking sex. I suggested they have sex three times a week all month long, with it being fairly evenly spread out (e.g., not going more than two days without intercourse).

They also needed to track *exactly* when Faith was fertile using the FAM guidelines for monitoring cervical mucus changes and an ovulation timing test, such as those by First Response™ or Fairhaven Health. During Faith's fertile time as indicated by either the presence of egg white cervical mucus (EWCM) or a positive ovulation test, they needed to have sex every other day (and it could be every day if they wanted). Also they needed to close out the babymaking with one "late session" within 24 hours of the *end* of Faith's EWCM, in case she was a late ovulator.

To Dan's great joy, I told them that sexual positions don't matter because sperm will reach the Fallopian tube within minutes after ejaculation no matter what they do as long as it includes penile-vaginal penetration. But, as I explained, what did matter for making the best sperm was that Dan be turned on during this fertile, babymaking sex. He should choose the positions they used during his orgasm. It needed to be hot for dad—he needed this and deserved it. I also suggested that they watch something sexy together in a video or pull out the lingerie and blindfolds at least once during

Faith's fertile time, again to increase dad's stimulation and sperm production. Happily, Dan and Faith did conceive their daughter several months after they started the "program."

Unfortunately, I didn't have Pre-Seed available yet when I met with Dan and Faith, but now my pep talk for couples in this situation also includes using Pre-Seed to optimize the environment for sperm and to help everyone find greater pleasure in their efforts to add to their family.

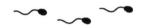

Infertility is far more common than most of us realize. One in five couples will have trouble conceiving and almost all of us know someone who has gone through this life challenge. Keep in mind that, in general, couples have about a 20% chance of conceiving each month, and approximately 80% of women will conceive in their first six months of unprotected intercourse. But when couples haven't gotten pregnant after this six-month window, a fertility evaluation is needed. And for women 35 or over that appointment should be scheduled after four months of trying to conceive, so they actually see someone by that six-month mark.

These initial fertility exams will rule out the four main causes of infertility. You can learn more about these as well as finding tips to improve natural conception rates at *SexScienceandNature.com*. In brief, three out of four couples who are not conceiving will have one of the following problems: 1) poor sperm quality; 2) abnormal ovulation or cycles; 3) Fallopian tube pathology; or 4) improperly timed intercourse. For insight into improving natural fertility, coupled with excellent medical advice, I suggest the books *A Baby At Last* by Rosenwaks, Goldstein and Fuerst; *Making Babies* by

David and Blakeway; or *Perfect Hormone Balance for Fertility: The Ultimate Guide to Getting Pregnant* by Greene and Tarkan.

As an andrologist, I would be remiss if I missed the opportunity to clarify that a diagnosis of male factor infertility should not be given based on one sperm sample reviewed solely by a laboratory. This diagnosis requires two sperm analyses using World Health Organization standards with collection occurring between two and four weeks apart. If a first semen sample is normal, the second test doesn't need to be done. But for men with abnormal sperm on an initial sperm sample, the second round of testing should be done to confirm poor sperm quality. If male factor issues are found during this testing, seek out a male reproductive specialist for ongoing care. These can be found by contacting the American Society of Andrology or the Society for Male Reproduction and Urology.

Why Waiting for a Baby is Risky

Fertility *dramatically declines* with age for both men and women. For women, this downward trend starts around thirty. In fact, fertility rates of 35-year-old women are *half* of that found in women in their early twenties. Miscarriage rates also begin to increase for women after 30. Even if a woman chooses not to have another child again for a few years, having that first baby before 35 gains the woman some time reproductively. This 35-year mark is of course a statistical average. Some women will have a drop in their fertility before this age. Therefore, if having kids is very important to an individual woman, 35 is the *latest* she should wait to conceive her first baby.

Male fertility also starts to decrease sometime in a man's 40s. And with all things sperm, it is the DNA that starts to degenerate first. Some studies have suggested a link between older fathers and negative outcomes in offspring, including miscarriages and childhood diseases. For men interested in fathering children later in life, getting the SCSA DNA test done prior to babymaking is a good idea to see if a few months of sperm tune-up (as in Dan's program) are needed.

Overall, no amount of wishful thinking will change our biologic reproductive aging patterns. And contrary to what many people think, assisted reproduction technology, such as in vitro fertilization, doesn't provide an automatic pass to avoid dealing with this issue. Most of us overestimate the number of babies born each year in the U.S. from ART as well as the success rate of these procedures. For context, around 4 million babies are born each year in the U.S. During the most recently measured year (2012), 165,000 in vitro fertilization procedures were done, resulting in **62,000 babies** being born. This figure represents the highest number of ART children born in a year. But it is still only 1.5% of American births. We must always remember and remind our legislators and medical experts that this means 98.5% of all American babies are conceived the good old-fashioned way of sperm meeting egg inside mommy's Fallopian tubes. The fertility struggles of millions of couples would benefit greatly from improved funding for research into methods to improve *natural* human reproduction.

Equally important to note in the above statistics, *most* in vitro procedures do *not* result in a baby. Waiting until we are older to conceive is not like deciding to have LASIK eye surgery. You don't "go in and have it done." ART is a treatment of last resort for people who cannot conceive naturally, and in two out three cycles, it will not work. We all need to know these numbers to help those around us make the best choices when they are staging the timing of the competing aspects of their lives (e.g., parenting versus careers).

Writing this, I think about my second cousin Hannah who called me about a year ago in incomprehensible tears. "My FSH is too high," she sobbed, and my heart sank. Hannah is a lawyer at a large U.S.

cosmetic company. She doesn't share her private life at work, but she is gay. At 43 when she called me, she had also been without a partner for the past five years. When she and Robin broke up, I asked Hannah, then 38, what she was thinking about kids. She told me, "I've got time to find the right person to parent with!" But I was worried that she would not stop (before it was too late) to map out what she wanted from the concept of "family." Now years later she had called me to let me know that even though she had decided to have a child as a single parent, her ovaries had gotten too old to form a normal egg. Hannah's chances of conceiving, even through IVF, were now less than 5%, and she would be hard-pressed to find a clinic to work with her given this reality. For women who are concerned that aging changes may be impacting their fertility, the First Response™ Fertility Test can detect hormone changes (such as Hannah had) showing a decrease in ovarian function and fertility.

For me personally, I was grateful I had Rayne when I was 33. I had developed a successful career, and I was at peace with my strengths and weaknesses in a way I hadn't been when I was younger. It was a blessing that I had an unplanned pregnancy which ended up being a very much wanted pregnancy. But now, approaching the age of 38 to conceive our second child was getting risky. I knew we needed to keep things moving forward.

Throughout this time I continued working to develop our AG-based fertility lubricant formula. Not only did other couples need it, but we needed it too! I was compounding and mixing various ingredients like a sorceress of old. Centrifuge tubes with different formulations, labeled with a black Sharpi, lay on lab counters and my desk at work, not to mention on the bathroom counters at home. I would mix a bit of this and that and then check the consistency between my fingers or on my forearm. If I liked the way the sample felt, I would have our technicians test it with sperm (to make sure it didn't harm them), and lastly, if all systems were "go," I would insert it inside myself with a syringe to see if it caused me any vaginal irritation. The cream of the cream, so to speak, then got used at home in real time (during intercourse) so we could note the slip and slide qualities of the different iterations—a tough job but someone had to do it.

After over half a year of trying to conceive, I became pregnant again. Everything with the pregnancy seemed fine until I was about sixteen weeks along and got into a minor fender bender. I was able to drive away after an exchange of information with the other driver. But that night as I lay on the couch, I started bleeding and felt like I was starting my period. Right away I called the doctor's office. When I went into the clinic for an ultrasound, the baby looked fine, but my bleeding didn't stop. After a few days, my medical training kicked in; I knew that if the bleeding continued, my pregnancy had a slim chance of surviving. There was no medical intervention that could be done. I just had to wait.

On the morning of the seventh day after the accident, I was showering when I looked down, and there was the placenta from my pregnancy lying near the drain. I screamed and Hank came running. Later, after being checked out, there seemed to be no medical reason for the loss. This baby girl had just decided to yield the right-of-way so that someone else could come along.

Mild Matters

After our loss, we took a break from TTC for a few months to let my uterus heal from the miscarriage. During this time, I continued the formulation research on our new fertility lubricant. I knew we would need to balance "toughness" and "mildness" to both protect sperm and provide great sex. During this time our lab, as well as others, was finally beginning to understand why leading lubricants were toxic to sperm. Specifically, we found that it was the ion concentration of the lubricants (i.e., their "salt" level), at up to 10 times the levels found in the semen and cervical mucus that sperm naturally swim in that was causing the damage. In fact, the lubricant induced sperm damage was equal to that seen for sperm in contact with contraceptive gels in laboratory testing. When sperm are exposed to solutions with these high salt concentrations, there is a rapid dehydration of water from inside the sperm, changing the cell shape (the cytoskeleton, for you biology buffs). This causes sperm membranes, tails and DNA to become structurally damaged, interfering with motility, capacitation and even embryo development if the sperm make it inside the egg.

As these reasons for sperm damage following contact with leading lubricants became clear, I knew our lubricant needed to be "isotonic": it would need to have the same ion concentration as semen and cervical mucus to provide sperm the optimal environment for their journey to the egg.

Radical Center Ruminations - Not surprisingly, since the discovery that high-ion concentration lubricants (many of the products on the shelf) harm sperm, it has since been reported that these same lubricants also damage the sensitive cells of intimacy. Specifically, they can harm the cells lining the woman's reproductive tract and the human rectum (impacted during anal intercourse in both men and women). By causing intimate cell sloughing (so that there is no longer an intact mucosal cell barrier), several common lubricants have been associated with an increased risk of sexual disease transmission.

Currently there is over a decade of work and at least 10 published studies showing the relationship between high osmolarity lubricants and intimate tissue damage, which may place users at possible risk for health problems including increased HIV transmission. Why aren't our national regulatory groups being much more aggressive in public health notifications on this topic? To my mind, if consumers knew the science they could more wisely choose when to use an isotonic lubricant, such as Pre-Seed.

I am proud to say that many of these same studies have looked at the Pre-Seed formula (also sold as Pre') and found it safe for the cells of intimacy. Although, of course, I would love it if everyone always used Pre-Seed as their lubricant, one can't help but ask why, given the body of science and our technological ability to make isotonic lubricants, high osmolarity lubricants continue to dominate our store shelves. Lubricant manufacturers and developers need to do better in bringing isotonic lubricants forward to enhance lovemaking without adding any risk to sex. Consumers, you need to demand this.

Slippery When Wet

Why do people use lubricants? Because when sex works the way it should, it is a slippery, wet affair. Sexual arousal of women causes the secretion of natural lubrication from cells in the vagina. These fluids make intercourse feel good for both partners. When women are aroused and become wet, the intensity of their sexual desire grows, leading to even more fluid production. When women are turned on, lovers exclaim "That makes me wet" or "You're so wet." Lubricants can shortcut the time needed for female arousal and/or supplement natural lubrication when it is in short supply, making sex comfortable and even more pleasurable for both the man and the woman.

As a reproductive physiologist, I was always intrigued by the concept that people put lubricants on the outside of the woman's vulva or on the man's penis. Neither of these are places that naturally have arousal fluid production! Topical skin application of a lubricant is good for helping ease the entrance of the penis into the vagina. But if things are still dry and tacky *inside* the vagina during intercourse, lubricants need to be reapplied or heavy duty products like oils and silicone (that can't be washed off easily and taste gross) are used. In either case, the lack of deep wetness and arousal throughout the vaginal canal doesn't feel as slippery or as spontaneous as natural arousal fluids.

While developing our fertility lubricant, I knew I wanted it to feel as natural as possible and therefore to be inserted deep inside the vagina to coat the walls of the vagina from the cervix to the vulva, just like a woman's arousal fluid. Our natural fluids evolved where they needed to be, and I trusted nature's choice on this. A slippery vaginal canal feels sexy to us. This internal lubrication makes for fun foreplay, as well as better intercourse, as fingers and the penis can stroke in and out and against our full clitoral area. As we designed our lubricant, following human sexual physiology seemed like the best choice to help women feel ready and turned on sooner and more intensely. And nothing turns a man on like the woman he loves being wet and ready for him, whether the couple is babymaking or lovemaking.

In addition to wanting our lubricant to be applied differently than most, I realized we also needed to change how we chose the ingredients for our product. We would start with what sperm needed.

I knew that if we identified a formula that was safe for sperm, it would almost certainly be safe for the intimate tissues of the human body (e.g., deep inside the vagina) since sperm are the human bodies' most fragile cells. Of course, AG would be on the list of ingredients we used because of its unique antioxidant capacity and the protection it provides for sperm.

To help us identify what else should be in this fertility formula, I reached out to Dr. David Mortimer, one of the foremost andrologists in the world. David has helped draft guidelines for the World Health Organization to define what "normal" sperm look like and has written leading textbooks on male reproduction. I knew he could tell me what our parameters needed to be for an ideal product that wouldn't harm sperm. After meeting with David, we decided that the lubricant should mimic as closely as possible the fertile cervical mucus made by a woman at ovulation.

A Good Kind of Mucus

Egg white cervical mucus or EWCM as it is known in TTC circles is nature's original sperm-safe lubricant. Mucus is an unflattering word, so much so that many people call these secretions "cervical fluids." Each month, as a woman nears ovulation, her ovary creates high levels of estrogen that enter her blood stream and bathe her cervical mucus glands causing a change in the make-up of these secretions. Normally, when estrogen is low, the cervical mucus is scant in quantity, thick and whitish and is made up of a mish-mash of overlapping microscopic fibers with a low pH that block sperm from swimming efficiently through the cervix. But during ovulation, suddenly, "ooo la la"…this mucus becomes the sperm's road to paradise! The estrogen changes the sugars in the cervical fibers so that they draw in high quantities of water. This forces the mucus fibers apart to form a highway that the sperm can swim up to reach the Fallopian tube. While normally having a low pH of less than 6, during ovulation cervical mucus pH rises to match that of semen (pH 7 to 8), which is of course the *exact pH* sperm need to best function so they can reach the Fallopian tube. The sugars and the water that come into the cervical mucus during ovulation increase the volume of mucus by more than ten-fold, thus widening and expanding the road the sperm travel on up through the vagina.

These changes result in the slippery, stretchy, clear mucus referred to as "egg white" cervical mucus because it looks like egg whites. Knowledgeable TTC women seek the magical EWCM like their fertility Holy Grail because it facilitates natural conception. It is the stuff the rest of us briefly note on our panties or on toilet tissue when we wipe a few days a month. It is nature's perfect lubricant and ideal for sperm, without it they would be stopped at the (cervical) gate and unable to reach the tubes and the egg.

Some women don't make this fertile EWCM, their bodies thus thwarting the ability of their partner's sperm to swim through the cervix of these gals. These women are said to have "hostile cervical mucus," a condition occurring in at last 15% of women. Most commonly, this occurs as women age, have hormone imbalances or take fertility medications, such as Clomid (the leading fertility prescription).

I knew that if we could make a lubricant that mimicked fertile cervical mucus secretions we would have a product that optimized fertility. But I was soon to realize that these same virtues of mildness and natural feeling in a lubricant could help women and couples who weren't trying to conceive as well.

Chapter 11

The Sacrifices We Make

Research was moving full steam ahead—on Fallopian tubes and sperm at the university and on our lubricant at the company. At the same time, however, I had two friends go through sexual-life crises that would help me think even further "outside the box" regarding our product development. Without these cases in my life, I may not have fully explored the need for a nonirritating lubricant product for use by *any* couple, not just those who were trying to conceive.

Angel, a good friend of mine in vet school, called one evening. She sounded tired on the phone but asked if she could come for a quick visit. I recalled how during vet school Angel, a blonde Australian dynamo, had become pregnant from a one-night stand with Jeff, a nice man with whom she shared little in common. Because they had both grown up Catholic, they married. Their adorable daughter was now 13 years old.

When Angel arrived, I saw that she was depressed and despondent. As we walked along the Spokane River, she told me that Jeff never seemed to care if they had sex or not. Angel felt that she was always the one who had to initiate intimacy, even though it only occurred once a month or so and usually left her unfulfilled. In fact, she told me she had only had an orgasm a few times with Jeff over the ten years of their marriage. Several times, recently, Jeff had walked in on her masturbating in their bathroom as she sought sexual release. This was of course humiliating for both of them.

"I don't know what God wants from me," she said in tears as we sat on a log by the water's edge. "Am I supposed to live and die this lonely?"

While I couldn't answer her deeper spiritual questions, I asked Angel if she and Jeff had ever tried a lubricant to at least make the sex they were having more enjoyable for her.

"Are you kidding?" she responded. "That would involve talking about sex...something we don't do, ever! Mostly, I wish we could make each other just feel good occasionally in our marriage, even if we aren't in love." I felt deeply sympathetic as I thought about ways to help Angel and women like her.

In the synchronicity of life, during this same month another friend, Tessa, called me. Tessa's husband, Chris, was also an andrologist and worked in the federal government studying the effects of chemicals on sperm. Chris and I were members of a self-proclaimed informal science and drinking group called the "Sperm Mafia," with goals (when we were sober) of ensuring high quality science at meetings and conferences in the field of sperm research. At our last get-together, I had mentioned my lubricant research, and Chris apparently had shared this with Tessa.

In her call to me now, she told me that her recent recovery from uterine cancer was wreaking havoc on her sex life. She, like many other pelvic cancer survivors, was having vaginal spasms in which her pelvic floor would tighten and close making vaginal penetration by her husband almost impossible. The spasms would cause pain for her, even during orgasm. "How unfair is that!" she laughed.

As we talked further, it became clear that the chemotherapy had damaged the cells in her body that made natural lubrication. But also her tissues were so thin and sensitive that she couldn't use commercial lubricants. "I tried olive oil," Tessa said, "but I got a terrible yeast infection afterwards. Honestly, sometimes I just give Chris a BJ so we don't have to deal with my "issues" all the time, but then I feel angry that he had a release and I didn't."

After she shared her situation, we discussed some ideas and then she asked me about my work. When I told her about my home testing on our newest lubricant prototypes, she remarked, "You know, since it won't kill sperm, it will probably be nonirritating to cancer survivors like me." Her observation sent my mind into yet another area in which a good lubricant could "change the world." If disease survivors like Tessa could use it, how great would that be! "I want to try some of your new lube," Tessa said, confirming my thoughts. I promised to have a compounding pharmacist mix our latest version for her. Within a week, I sent it to her so she could try it out. Tessa and Chris loved the Pre-Seed prototype!

Angel and Tessa made me think a lot about the larger context of sexuality in our human relationships and how a carefully designed lubricant that optimized cell function and honored our body's own natural physiology might be useful for many more people than we had first envisioned.

Humans, by their very DNA and biology, are sexual. But as with everything in life, there is a bell curve in people's baseline for sexual desire. A few people are outliers, having very low or very high levels of desire for sex, but most people are average. These normal (average) people make up the large cup shape of the bell, and the outliers make up the bell's flared outer edges. Our inherent sexual drive is individually unique based largely on the amount of sex steroids our body makes (e.g., levels of estrogen and testosterone). We can well imagine a benefit for human communities to have a mix of people with high and low sex steroids and, therefore, high and low levels of sexual desire. In other words, a bell curve is good. Our ancestors needed people who "lived for sex" in order to keep procreation of the species going, even through fighting, famine and floods; yet they also needed people who would prioritize hunting for food or inventing a new spear over having sex. Most of the people in these early villages had a normal amount of sex, but that didn't make either the high or low outliers in the group "bad," "wrong," or "abnormal" in a pathological sense. Sex was sex, and people had sex as much as they needed, wanted or could get within their social hierarchy.

When humans brought culture, marriage and religion into the equation, things changed. Instead of a person with a high sex drive seeking out a willing partner to fulfill their sexual need at the moment, now two people who were contractually partnered had to negotiate each other's different sexual desire levels *for life!* Often, inevitably, one or the other of the couple might have sexual needs that were outside of the larger bell part of average human sexual desire while the other partner was more average. This, of course, was a recipe for conflict.

When One of You Wants Sex and the Other Doesn't

Angel and Jeff, like millions of other couples, suffered from *sexual discrepancy.* It can manifest in different levels of need or desire for sexual activity between two partners and in different levels of sexual satisfaction for the two parties (within the sex they do have). Much of sexual discrepancy between the two halves of a whole couple is, at its foundation, genetic or DNA-based and is an expression of the differing hormone levels between the individuals that make up the pair. This is important to realize so that we don't consider our partner "messed up" or ourselves as flawed or "bad" if our partner is less or more sexually excitable or interested than we are. At the same time, sexual discrepancy can also be a result of emotional, relational and physical difficulties in the pair-bond. In Tessa's case, her cellular disease had created sexual discrepancy. In Angel and Jeff's case, relational and emotional issues in many areas of their life were most likely causing significant sexual issues that were decreasing their sexual satisfaction.

Sexual satisfaction—the most easily treatable part of sexual discrepancy—is our feeling of pleasure, joy and excitement (without anxiety or negative stress) during intimacy. In most cases, you and your partner can work on sexual satisfaction even if other parts of the marriage are floundering. This is very important work because research from around the world reveals that sexual satisfaction is highly related to overall relationship satisfaction and thus marital longevity. If the two individuals' sexual needs are satisfied, the couple will tend to stay together longer and/or will have a more satisfying marriage, even if they don't have textbook-perfect communication skills or tend to fight frequently. In short, good sex can make up for other flaws in the relationship.

Talking with Angel later that spring afternoon of her visit, with the sun coming through our living room window, I felt that she and Jeff had never been given the tools to try to "find themselves sexually" within their marriage. They had not looked at or talked about their sexual discrepancies or what provided sexual satisfaction. From what Angel was describing, it sounded like Jeff was having "compliant sex." He didn't really want to be having sex with Angel but said "yes" out of a sense of duty. He was not too unusual in this regard: studies show that 55-65% of women and 35-40% of men have said yes to sex they didn't want during marriage. And during a two-week window in one study, 50% of women and 26% of men consented to compliant sex at least once. There is nothing wrong with this in a partnership; it is part of the compromise that keeps a marriage strong.

But when sex is only or mostly the compliant type for one member in a couple, the bonds of the relationship will weaken. Sex is, literally, a glue (think of the fluids transferring between you as physical, spiritual and emotional glue) that helps relationships survive and flourish. If you are feeling some kind of sexual compliance as a constant in your relationship or are feeling sexual discrepancy or low sexual satisfaction of any significant kind, it is crucial to talk about it, as scary as that can be.

Sexual Discrepancy

Sexual desire discrepancy in marriage occurs when one partner has an internal disagreement between their desire and the actual sexual frequency they are experiencing. And remember, sexual discrepancy isn't just about how often a couple has sex. It is also about what sex acts they share and the level of satisfaction each of them feels during the sex. Thus, it is about both quantity and quality. In recent studies, individuals in marriage who wished to experience different sex acts *more often* than they were actual getting them (such as men who wanted more oral sex) and those who wished to experience certain sex acts significantly *less often* than they were (such as women who wanted less anal sex) were both more likely to be dissatisfied with their relationships.

Overall, the research shows that men have more unmet needs between desired and actual sexual frequency than women, with 41%

of men versus 22% of women expressing a high discrepancy in not getting enough of what they want over an extended time frame. For males, high sexual discrepancy and lack of frequency can result in low sexual satisfaction that can make the man feel more negative about the relationship as a whole.

In spite of the prevalence of sexual "disconnect," some couples get it right and are a good match in sexual desire, with 37% of individuals reporting no sexual discrepancy with their partner. But this number also means that *most* couples feel some kind of discrepancy. Fortunately, for many of these couples, the discrepancy is not significant; but for Angel and Jeff, the discrepancy was dangerous to their already weak pair-bond. Although Jeff was having compliant sex with Angel to avoid conflict with her, it wasn't satisfying her needs either. Because Angel and Jeff never even mentioned that something was going on, there was no talk, loud or soft, about the poor quality of their sex. In light of these dire circumstances, we needed a dramatic intervention to move this couple somewhere new, for better or for worse, so they could figure out their future together.

In order to begin this intervention, Angel needed to be armed with some knowledge of what was within the range of normal for human sexual relationships. She also needed the courage to share and ask more for what she wanted during sex…and she needed to be very open to hearing what Jeff needed too.

What Do You Want?

It is completely normal to want more or less of something in our intimate relationships than what we are experiencing. In fact, you can compare what you would like to change about your sex life with data from a study involving 10,000 people between the ages of 33 and 43. In this study, the researchers found the following:

- People wanted to kiss or make out four to six times a week but were only kissing two to three times a week. Surprisingly, more than half of both men and women wanted more kissing, so it wasn't just women who wanted this.

- Among men, 81% wanted more oral sex, 75% wanted more vaginal sex and 47% wanted more anal sex.

- Among women, 48% wanted more vaginal sex, 36% wanted more oral sex and very few (8%) wanted more anal sex.

Anal sex was the least favored activity for both sexes, with men wanting it less than once a month and most women fine with "not at all."

Interestingly, the sex act men were *most* satisfied with was their solo masturbation. Of the guys, 53% were satisfied with the amount they were doing it, but almost a third *wanted to be doing less of it* (in other words, they would have preferred good sex with a partner to masturbation). Only 15% of women wanted to be masturbating more or less than they were.

An interesting twist in this study showed up in how higher desires for certain activities impacted overall relationship satisfaction. Wanting more kissing and vaginal intercourse was associated with higher satisfaction in the partnership for both men and women (likely these couples enjoyed their nookie time). In contrast, for both men and women, wanting more masturbation was negatively associated with relationship satisfaction. If sex felt better alone than with the partner, things were not going well in the couple.

Interestingly, a higher desire for anal intercourse for the man was also associated negatively with relationship satisfaction, as was the desire for more sexual fantasies in women. It seems to make sense that couples who enjoy making love with each other and who know how to please each other want more of the activities that have mutual interactions, such as kissing and vaginal intercourse, even while these couples know to mix things up with novelty, new positions, sex toys and other sex play.

We All Desire Sexual Desire

In another global study of 12,000 women and men, the most highly regarded aspect of sex was *feeling sexual desire for one's partner*. More than 70% of both men and women wanted this feeling (that is an extremely high and consistent number for biological science). The feeling of sexual desire for a partner was *more valued* than the actual physical feeling of pleasure itself during sex!

This speaks volumes about the instinctual level of sex and reproduction in our lives—we "need" to have sex to reproduce, and to have sex we need to feel desire. No matter how we dress it up, compliant sex just isn't that great. The saving grace here is that, especially for women, starting to have sex to comply with our partner's desire can *arouse* us, especially if time is taken in foreplay and in a well-written, well-rounded sexual script (such as the "Seven Stages of Foreplay" discussed in the next chapter). Desire can then jump out and take both partners by surprise. In my life, this usually looks like, "I am too tired. Don't worry about me tonight," then he starts fooling around and my attitude quickly changes to "Slow down, wait for me, I didn't mean it." This ends in fulfilling sex and orgasms for both of us.

In talking with Angel, I suggested she try the tried-and-true equation for better sex. One of the best ways to feel more desire is by increasing sexual frequency. People who have more sex generate higher levels of testosterone that in turn makes them want to keep having more sex. This is a very good thing because people (both men and women) who feel higher levels of sexual desire in their relationships have fewer thoughts of ending their current relationship and starting a new one. And given that a majority of people (58% of women and 57% of men) are *not satisfied* with their sex lives, and 24% of women and 36% of men have less sex than they want, the only real failsafe for positively affecting our sexual chemistry is to have more sex...and to prioritize making it more varied and playful.

Angel saw the wisdom of my advice as we shared, but she also had to think realistically about how many times a week she and Jeff might have sex. Normally, for reproductive-aged people having sex two to three times a week is one of the best ways to keep the home fires burning. But Angel and I agreed that baby steps were required for her and Jeff. For them, the goal of once a week might be sufficient for them to grow in their skills together and to foster better intimacy.

Don't Forget Quality!

Increasing your *quantity* of sex is a biochemical way of keeping passions going, but, of course, the *quality* of your sex life matters a lot as well. As Angel and I talked, I kept thinking there must be something else going on with Angel and Jeff that still wasn't clear from our discussions. So I asked her to explain the "sexual script" she and Jeff followed. Their script boiled down to this: Angel would make a bid in the dark by touching Jeff on the arm. He would then roll over on top of her and kiss her lightly, never passionately. Within a few minutes he would grab his erect penis and spread her legs a bit to thrust into her, using saliva if things were dry. After four to five minutes of thrusting, Jeff would come in silence, roll off of Angel and head to their shared bathroom to clean up. Sex always involved the missionary position and was always soundless. Because she followed this script with Jeff only about 10 to 12 times a year, Angel didn't have much chance to even try small things to change up the quality of their intimacy.

In helping Angel analyze the couple's sexual script, I reminded her that the sounds mammals make before and during sex (including the human voice and language) are part of the physiology that triggers desire. They are "sexy" to our partners. We discussed that it would be useful to try to do some talking during or around sex. Although many married couples are restricted by insecurity or fear in how they talk about sex and during it, research shows that guys, not surprisingly, often get off on crude talk around sex. Men report a greater use of terms such as tits, pussy, cock and clit than women during sex. Surprisingly, there is also a significant relationship between the frequency of using these types of words and relational satisfaction and closeness for both men and women. The ability to openly discuss sexual matters with slang terms can create an ease of sharing between the partners that is associated with better sexual satisfaction.

As Angel thought about ways to vocalize during sex, I knew she wasn't about to start screaming, "Fuck me harder!" when she got home. But she seemed to be clear on a plan of action in which she would at least tell Jeff she "wanted him" when she would touch his arm or vocalize a "That feels good" when he would kiss her even slightly more intensely. She would do this, she decided, both to arouse them both more and also in a subtle bid to slow him down during intercourse so she could come.

Also I asked her to let go of her anger about always being the one who had to initiate sex between them. Not having sex wasn't going to fix their problems, and it appeared that Jeff wasn't going to start asking for it any time soon, so for a while at least, she would most likely need to continue being the initiator.

Who Should Initiate Sex?

Sexual desire and initiating sex are, of course, linked. In one study of younger couples, only 23% of women and 10% of men *never* initiated sex during a one-week slice of married life, suggesting that both genders usually take turns in this role. That said, on average, men more often ask for sex—in part due to our ancient mating strategy differences but also partly due to our social expectations. Among college-aged couples, 38% of women thought men should initiate sex more than women, but only 16% of men thought this was right (guys want to feel wanted too!).

Although it is well within the range of normal in a relationship for one partner to initiate sex more than the other, taking turns giving the hint or asking the question will often heat things up and can help each partner feel pursued. Personally, I feel a bit slighted if I have to initiate "getting busy" too many times without hubby taking the lead. For me, if I am asking more than three times in a row, I feel like I am somehow not desirable enough for him to go out on a limb for some action. And, guys, you can't say, "She knows I always want it, so it's up to her to initiate it." That's not an excuse for you not to make your wife feel wanted. You should both *noticeably* take the lead now and then. Asking for sex is a risky, vulnerable act even if you have been together forever. Honor that.

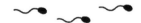

Angel promised to keep me apprised as to whether after two or three months of trying to make some sexual changes with Jeff, he might initiate sex once in a while. We decided that holding that goal in mind might be a good way of trying to "test" whether the new strategies were working. We thought that if Jeff started initiating sex even once in a while, the couple's marriage might improve on many levels.

As Angel and I wrapped up our "girls' time," I reached in my pocket and handed her some of the Pre-Seed prototype that I had had mixed recently. The lubricant product sat inside sealed sterile syringes. As she put them away for safekeeping, I gently told her, "Angel, I don't know what all is going on with Jeff, but put this in your vagina half an hour before you plan to launch project 'I want you' and let me know how it goes."

Several weeks later Angel called me sounding much stronger and more certain than before. She explained how using our lubricant inside her vagina had made her feel wet, and then when Jeff slid his penis (I think she said cock!) along her clitoris, she felt excited and grabbed his wrist to guide him to keep doing the motion. This quickly brought her to orgasm! The lubrication and lack of "dry sex" actually made Jeff last longer inside of her, and she had another orgasm during intercourse ("the first time in a long time," she smiled over the phone!).

Things weren't magically fixed between her and Jeff, but they were better. Over the next year, Angel and Jeff developed enough language around sex that he could share his heart. In fact, one day he confessed the "deeper issue" in the sexual relationship: he was and always had been gay. He hadn't wanted to hurt Angel or their daughter, and he had tried with everything in himself to be "in love" with his wife. He apologized for his lack of honesty, saying he realized now that by hiding his true sexual self, he wasn't just harming himself but also Angel.

When I spoke to Angel about this she started crying, but her words sounded almost hopeful: "It wasn't me, I understand now it wasn't something wrong with me." This was a bittersweet realization, but Angel's voice revealed a new sense of self-confidence. I didn't know at the time but have since learned that Angel's situation is not uncommon. There are an estimated two to three million straight spouses in past or present marriages with bisexual, gay or lesbian partners. To better understand mixed-orientation marriages, read James Oliver Chapman's *How to Lose Your Wife to Another Woman* and seek out the Straight Spouse Network (*straightspouse.org*) if you need support.

Madame Curie and Me

As I got positive feedback from both Angel and Tessa that the lubricant formulation was helping them at home, I also continued testing in the lab and at my home. Finally, on one of our last ski trips of the season, all the stars (and the lube and the sperm and the egg) aligned for conception of my second son, more than five years after our first. Sage Torbin (who would later add a "y" to his name to become Sayge) was born at 12 p.m. on December 12, 1997 after a 12-minute labor! Some unknown Resident at Deaconess Hospital ran into my room to catch Sayge on his way out, with no time for my doctor to make it.

Sayge was busy in utero during my pregnancy and has stayed that way ever since! As a newborn, he was too distracted by life and all that was going on around him to do anything as boring as nurse. To feed him I had to lie down on our bed in the dark. This was head-bangingly boring for me—I couldn't read or even move for many hours per day if I wanted him to reliably feed. This was not part of my second child "fantasy." But life has always been fun with Sayge around!

After having produced the classic heir and a spare in children, I still had one last task to participate in before hanging up my reproductive tract. Because I still had Fallopian tubes, I could be the one to answer a burning question in my scientific field. But more on that later... first, here's a little background.

By the time Sayge was born in 1997, the attachment of sperm to Fallopian tube cells in other species had been well described in several publications, from my own in graduate school to that of others. The specifics of this sperm attachment to the animal FT cells had been studied using scanning electron microscopes (SEM) that provided beautiful images of stallion or bull sperm with their long tails streaming behind them, "held" tightly against the FT cells from a mare or cow, respectively. The long finger-like cilia of the tubal cells could be seen wrapping around the sperm, holding them snuggly to their surface (acting like the seat belts for our sperm passengers in our plane metaphor).

Still other detailed photos came from transmission electron microscopy (TEM). This technology showed the "ultrastructure" of the sperm and tubal cells. Unlike an SEM, with its view of cells from afar like an airplane flying over a landscape, TEM shows a slice through the cells like taking a cross section through a mountain and looking at all the different rock layers that make up the mountain. With the TEM photos, we could see that sperm and FT cells' membranes became so closely joined during the sperm's nurturing stage (when they attached to the tubal cells) that it was literally impossible to always see two separate cells (that of the individual sperm and that of the individual tubal cells). In fact, the two types of cells appeared functionally joined together as one to aid in the transfer of sugars and other factors from the FT cells to the sperm.

Although we had these amazing pictures for animal tissues, we had not yet shown that human sperm and FT cells worked this way. Even though my lab could grow human Fallopian tube cells in a Petri dish by collecting them from women and culturing them and although I had gotten some nice photos of human sperm attaching to these FT cells in the system, neither of these steps *proved* that sperm were naturally stored in the woman's FT in the same manner as seen in other species (the "burning" question). With other species, we could breed an ovulating female and a few hours later surgically remove her tubes to study sperm interactions with the FT, but we could not do this experiment in humans, neither ethically nor logistically. However, there was one way I could see how sperm were stored in a woman's Fallopian tubes—and that was if I did the experiment on myself!

I decided that I had "but one set of tubes to give" and made plans to give it. Luckily, my amazing and equally curious Ob-Gyn (Dr. Lori Smetana) was willing to sit down with me to map out a plan for an alteration to the tubal sterilization surgery I had intended to have done when Sayge was six months old. Painstaking care would be required during this surgery as she would need to be able to preserve the tube's structure *and* remove as much of my tube as possible for study. We designed the experiment to include intercourse the morning before surgery to get hubby's sperm to the tubes before they were removed. Because I was still breastfeeding, I wasn't ovulating (remember ovulation makes the sperm-protecting FT sugars). Dr. Smetana helped out by putting me on estrogen pills to mimic the changes in increasing estrogen levels that would normally occur in a women's body when she was ready to ovulate.

The week before the surgery, I asked Dr. Christine Davitt, the supervisor of the Electron Microscopy Lab at Washington State University, to send up all the specialized vials and preservatives needed to fix (secure) the tissues so that she could later make the small slices for the EM imaging. We knew we only had one shot—there was no "do over" if we got it wrong. Also, because I would be sound asleep during the procedure, we had to have every step lined up in advance; I wouldn't be available to help my team troubleshoot while I was under anesthesia.

I was so excited the night before the surgery that I could barely sleep. What if I was wrong and Hank's sperm did not interact with my tubal cells at all? In this case, all my hypotheses would be wrong, and the overall thrust of my research for the past ten years would prove incorrect! What if the sperm and tubal interactions were messed up because I wasn't ovulating? Did I hold the right physiologic potential for this experiment (being a breastfeeding mom rather than a fertile woman)? But science is all about risk-taking and follow-through, so I just had to believe we were doing the right thing. I also knew I would have to wait in anticipation for about a month while Dr. Davitt completed and sent back the study images.

The next morning, we did "the deed" before the boys woke up. I had to focus on having an orgasm so that I could be absolutely sure that the transport of hubby's sperm to my tubes was "optimized." Then I headed to the hospital. Dr. Smetana came into the pre-op room with the routine surgery forms for me to sign. Then less routinely, she and I went over the different specimen containers she would place the Fallopian tubes in after she had removed them from my body. After a warm blanket and an IV injection…the next thing I remember was feeling peaceful for a moment then drifting back into consciousness. Suddenly I jolted wide awake, excitedly asking, "Did you get it, did you get it!?" Dr. Smetana smiled proudly, holding up the plastic specimen containers holding my floating Fallopian tubes, the very tissue my children had begun their lives in. Dr. Davitt's courier then rushed in to carry my tubes back down to WSU's expert laboratory. "Goodbye…fingers crossed!" I thought as my tubes left the building in a foam container on ice.

Although I was very busy with an infant and my research labs, I waited like a nervous hen to hear and see what Dr. Davitt's group would find. Finally, a few weeks later, I saw the caller identification message of "WSU EM Lab" as the phone rang at my desk. My hands almost shook as I answered. "Joanna," Chris said, "They are there!" I covered my mouth with my hand, and tears sprang to my eyes. As any lay person would assume (given that we are mammals just like other species)—but against much of the teaching of the medical community at that time—*human sperm did attach to the Fallopian tube cells in women,* just like they did in other species!

Chris kept talking and it took me a moment to understand her as she said, "I am faxing you photos right now." Excitedly I told her I would call back later and ran to our office fax machine. There, unfolding, were EM photos of my husband's sperm intimately attached to my Fallopian tube cells, exactly as I had seen in the cow and mare research I had done before. It was breathtaking and cause for a celebratory dinner with my family!

Chapter 12

All Business All The Time

As my NIH research was coming to a conclusion and final manuscripts and reports were being drafted, across town at the company lab it was becoming obvious that if we were going to successfully launch a fertility lubricant we needed money, major money. But between doing my research at WSU, being CEO of the company and mothering two kids with only part-time childcare, my life was becoming a "no time to pee" type of busy. Even evenings and weekends would find me at my home computer completing data analysis and write-ups. Hank was able to change his hours during this time so that he could pick up more of the childcare. But we routinely worked opposite hours to take care of our sons. In the end, all this work paid off with the company receiving more than eight U.S. and international patents, but the stress became an integral part of our marriage. Hank and I felt little romance. We kept having sex, but it became pretty locked into the "known knowns" that worked to bring pleasure easily and quickly in our hectic lives. We had begun the relationship stage of little romance, functional sex and drifting intimacy.

During this time, it became clear that if the business was going to grow, we were going to need to bring in investment dollars. For that I realized I would have to continue my over-extended schedule, deal with my fear of public speaking and endure sleepless road-warrior nights away from my kids as I began traveling with our "dog and pony show" pitching our technology to potential investors. I would soon learn that most of these meetings took on a familiar pattern— me, a petite, blonde woman, having breakfast or lunch with three or four men who were fifteen to twenty years older than me, talking about vaginal secretions and semen. Many men (and these potential investors were over 98% men) would smirk during our discussions or make a truly enlightened comment like, "I've never used a lubricant in my life. I can't imagine why you would need one unless you're bad in bed." These comments would then turn the meeting into a raucous debate over the merits of vaginal lubricants in general rather than looking at the actual need for *our* fertility lubricant.

Repeatedly I was told there simply was not a market for this product—until the meeting was done. As I was leaving, almost without exception, someone would ask, "Dr. Ellington, do you have a moment?" Outside the restaurant or around the corner from colleagues, I would hear story after story from top businessmen and industry leaders about their own struggles with infertility: tears and years of trying to conceive, broken hearts, broken dreams and broken relationships.

"Please, can you get my wife and me some of your lubricant to try?" they would ask. Yet outside of my carefully selected friends and me, Pre-Seed wasn't ready for people to be using at home. I felt sad that I had to let them know they would need to wait a bit longer for our product.

Nearing my fortieth birthday, I knew things were not going well on many fronts in my life. I was out of shape and overweight. Hank and I rarely saw each other and when we did, we seemed to have little in common. I had recently taken a quiz in one of Dr. Phil's books and identified that we were "emotionally" divorced. Although I shared the test results with Hank, we ran out of time to discuss it; one of the boys had the flu, and I had some new data on a lubricant prototype I needed to analyze before flying to Houston for a pitch the next day.

I remember, on the night of my birthday, our friends called to see if we wanted to go celebrate the big 4-0 and I said "no." I was too tired. Instead I drew a bath in our soaker tub and then let it slowly drain all the way around me. I felt too tired to even get out of the chilling water left in the bottom of the tub as I pondered if my life would ever be anything but overworked and full of drudgery. I had two brilliant, entertaining children. I had gained professional respect with my research and publishing. But a breakthrough technology to help infertile couples was stalled for lack of funding and the right business knowledge on my part. Also, with my marriage in serious trouble, I felt like I had limited potential for future success at home or at work and no time (or energy) to recharge my batteries.

I decided it was time for some intervention. Over the next few months, I started working out with a personal trainer, went on antidepressants and did hypnotherapy. The antidepressants gave me a side effect I hated—I couldn't orgasm—so those pills became a short-lived experiment. But I loved hypnotherapy with Dr. Jayne Helle in Spokane. After my visits with Jayne, I felt relaxed and capable, full of love and energy to give my kids. I began to realize that in distancing from their dad at home, I was also distancing from my children when I was there. Although I worked to make myself more present at home, in the end, several years later, this realization would be what would finally lead me to my second divorce: I absolutely did not want to become emotionally absent from my children as I had seen many other overworked, unhappy parents do.

Looking back, I don't know what I would have done differently to better control the chaos and severe emotional stress of those years that contributed to the end of my marriage. I don't know if I would not have made the AG discovery, or stopped the fertility lubricant development, or just thrown my hands up and quit my scientific work. There seemed to be no good choices during this "trapped" phase of my life except making sure I managed my time and energy with my kids as my top priority.

Running a Woman-Owned "Sex" Business

The year after my 40th birthday was a swirl of research at the University with a new grant looking at the damaging impact of antidepressants on sperm function. There was also the ever-present travel and meetings with prospective funding partners for the company. During these interactions, I met a local leader in Spokane, Mr. P, who supported regional biotechnology startups. Once a month he would host dinners at his home to which he invited different leaders (including state senators) for a fabulous meal and brainstorming session on how to help Spokane grow. After one of these dinners, I received a request from Mr. P's assistant to meet with him one-on-one; he wanted to learn about our company and the lubricant we were working on.

In the end, Mr. P decided to invest in our company, but as funding documents were being drawn up, I told our attorneys Jim Lisbakken and Erik Iverson with Perkins Coie in Seattle that I was nervous about receiving funding from Mr. P's venture capital division rather than from Mr. P himself as an "angel investor." Sometimes venture capitalists turn aggressive and try to take over the companies they invest in, hence their often cited nickname "Vulture Capital." As a result, Erik and Jim worked to make sure that the documents protected our company from future meddling by any new investors.

Along with investing cash, Mr. P offered us decreased rent for a beautiful windowed office in his downtown skyscraper. The new change in ownership of the company required changes in our corporate structure and a new name, BioOrigyn (or "Bio"). We also separated out a unique division for bringing the lubricant to market, "ING Fertility," named after the Nordic god of fertility, "Ing." With this new identity and a capital infusion, we were ready to get that fertility-friendly lubricant to market! We hired more staff to kick things into high gear, including my then housekeeper, Amy Gibson, who started as a file clerk for Bio and eventually worked up to become our office manager over the years. In the laboratory, Julie Schimmels moved from my WSU lab to head up Bio's research team. We were ready to finalize development and marketing strategies to launch our fertility lubricant.

One of our first jobs was to think of a name for this world's first fertility lubricant. Over the years we had tried out a few different names: "Enhance," "Pro-Cept" and JATO (my dad suggested this one, as in "Jet Assisted Take Off," an old WWII term). But none seemed quite right. One night, while working on the computer, I felt a growing energy inside me, literally a physical buzz in my chest, and then the phrase "Pre-Seed" came to mind. I typed the word out in Times New Roman font, size 16....Pre-Seed, a product that was applied "pre" (before) the "seed" (the sperm) came along. The next day I handed the typed sheet with this one name on it to several folks at work. One glance was all it took for everyone to agree: "That's it!"

The next task was identifying the right applicators for the product. We knew we wanted the fertility lubricant to be deposited inside the vagina where it could coat the internal vaginal walls and cervical opening with the optimal solution for sperm to swim through. But we still needed to identify the right kind of applicator to deliver the product to where we wanted it to be placed. To find the best delivery device, Amy was sent to the closest Rite Aid Pharmacy (which happened to be in the "Red Light" part of downtown Spokane) to buy anything she could find that was meant for insertion into the vagina or rectum. She filled a shopping cart with yeast treatments, douches, enemas—you name it! As she went to check out, the poor blushing male clerk triple-bagged all the items. "Don't worry," Amy quipped, "It's just for work." The clerk must have thought Amy was a prostitute with a lot of issues.

The TCOYF Gift

As we finalized package design and prepared to launch Pre-Seed, the product received one of those serendipitous endorsements that put it in front of millions of couples. In 2002, my baby sister, Elizabeth, was in medical school at the University of Washington preparing to be a gynecologist. Liz and I had both read Toni Weschler's book *Taking Charge of Your Fertility* (TCOYF) and used her methods in our own lives. One day Elizabeth suggested, "Why don't you call Toni and tell her about Pre-Seed?" Readers of Toni's bestselling books already knew that lubricants harmed sperm due to her excellent discussion of the subject in TCOYF.

Toni was warm and enthusiastic when I cold-called her. During the conversation, she asked if I would like to be a guest moderator at her very popular fertility internet chat-room (*TCOYF.com*). The next week I started a new "Q & A with Dr. E" at the website and began "meeting couples" (electronically) from diverse socio-economic groups. The women ranged from a military wife whose husband was coming home from his second tour in Afghanistan with a week to "get pregnant" before he left again to fundamentalist Christian, Jewish and Muslim women whose faiths did not allow them to use IVF. I also learned a lot about what fertility challenges look like from "inner city, low income, no insurance" vantages to those of the counterculture "granola" couple living off the grid near Taos, New Mexico. I realized that I, and the fertility industry as a whole, had a subconscious bias that somehow infertility in lower income or non-mainstream people didn't "really" matter. Yet it seemed like Pre-Seed could be a product that could benefit all kinds of couples.

Several months later as Pre-Seed was launching, Toni's new edition of TCOYF also hit the shelves. I was ecstatic to receive an autographed copy of the book from her with a note to check out her reference to Pre-Seed! In her bestselling book, Toni had written an updated lubricant section which discussed how commercial lubricants harm sperm—and also declared that fortunately there was now a lubricant, called "Pre-Seed," that didn't interfere with sperm function. With this announcement, her book introduced millions of readers to the concept of a "fertility-friendly" lubricant and to Pre-Seed itself.

Just in time (given Toni's mention of Pre-Seed in an international bestselling book), after years of dreaming and development, Pre-Seed was ready for the marketplace. Initially product sales were exclusively through *drugstore.com*, and within its first few months Pre-Seed became the number one selling product in their "medicine cabinet" category, with a 4.5 star rating! We found that people liked Pre-Seed so much (because it felt natural and had no bad taste) that they continued to use it even after they were done trying to conceive. Right away, we began receiving the outpouring of joyful Pre-Seed user stories that still make the Pre-Seed "Success Stories" page the most visited place at the product website. Our careful "birthing" of Pre-Seed had led to a very healthy product indeed...and we could not have been more proud!

Good Times, Bad Times

But as often happens in life, even within this incredibly exciting time of work bringing our new product to market, my personal life was going through its own landmark—and not a happy one. Once the funding came into Bio, late night hours at the company office became the norm. I needed this time to complete tasks that required deep concentration such as website development and package design. But in the dark night working in my office, I began to realize how much I was avoiding going home. Hank and I had become increasingly awkward together. Our unspoken words echoed between us, creating an expanding distance in our goals and dreams. The vibrancy, passion and fulfillment of the work I was doing with Pre-Seed contradicted with the lack of connection I felt at home. I wanted to be myself around my children and not just live tiptoeing around a failed relationship in their presence. Finally, I decided my best parenting would be outside of the marriage, not from within it.

Throughout the process of our divorce, we worked to create a co-parenting plan that honored each other's roles in our boys' lives. We developed a rotating two night-two night-three night joint custody schedule. This was tricky with our jobs, but it made sure neither parent was ever apart from the boys for more than three nights as we moved into a new definition of "family." Additionally, we sought to always sit next to each other at sporting events or concerts so that the boys didn't feel fragmented trying to "take care" of both parents during times when they should just be celebrating the victories in their lives.

Soon after this busy time of beginnings at work and endings at home, I fell in love again. In fact, I fell in love in one of those lightning bolt moments right out of a romance novel. Dr. Gilbert Dennis Clifton

(Gil), my present husband, was then a professor at Washington State University and entered into my life at one of Mr. P's dinners. I still recall seeing Gil standing in Mr. P's doorway in his black cashmere turtleneck, briefcase in his right hand, with the hall light casting a warm glow around him. I knew in that instant that I was going to end up spending the rest of my life with this man, even though I knew little about him at the time. In the deepest parts of my brain, I felt what every lover feels who has fallen in "love at first sight," the wash of pheromones, dopamine and oxytocin imprinting an image in the brain so profound and strong that it will remain forever etched in my mind and heart.

Over time Gil and I began blending our lives together in the many ways that grownups do when they have "real" jobs, kids and exes. Part of that blending involved writing a new sexual script with another adult. It was during this time with Gil that I finally and fully understood how important sexual scripts are for couples.

Pillow Talk

As adults in our forties, Gil and I both brought insights and experiences from life to our new relationship. We knew that our partnership needed to maintain a sense of priority, despite significant stresses in our family and professional lives. We also were aware that we needed to ask for what we wanted sexually in a clear, unequivocal way. And that sex is essential to passionate love. I did not realize at the time, but have since learned that good sex is a *leading indicator* of whether or not a relationship will last over time. But we all know sometimes it is hard to be clear in bed with another person when you aren't really sure about what you want yourself. Often the best sex takes reflection and a better understanding of what it is at the core that is making you turned off or turned on by something.

I have had thousands of people talk to me about sex over the years: teens, newlyweds, young parents in the thick of things, people in mid-life crisis, senior citizens, gay people, straight people and "I'm not sure people." I have discovered that when it comes to sex, there are five primary categories of people.

1) Partners who want to please you but don't know how.

2) Partners who care about pleasing you but not enough to overcome their laziness in bed.

3) Partners who once cared about pleasing you but have now given up.

4) Partners who are selfish and don't care what you ask for or need as long as what happens works for them.

5) Partners who do please you.

If you have a partner who pleases you sexually, take a moment to be grateful! Some of the rest are trainable and worth the effort, some are not.

Let's talk about an easy one first. With selfish partners, it is possible that no amount of talking, showing or exploring will help improve sex with them. These partners are the ones who verbally attack you when you express a desire for better sex for yourself. In the extreme, these people are physically violent and sexually abusive. Usually the right approach with this type of person is to leave them. These people can be men with heavy porn usage that gives them a sadistic or push-button approach to sex, or they can be women who think sex isn't worth the effort and chide their men for not loving them "in spite" of a sexless marriage.

That said the other types of people are statistically more common. For the first three types on my list, let's work backwards from #3 to #1. The folks in #3 are usually men who start out a relationship expecting the woman to orgasm and enjoy sex. If she is not able to over time, these men may just give up, feeling that the pressure to perform is undermining the intimacy or because they lack the confidence to determine what to do to improve things.

Behind Door #2 we have a lot of people, including myself at times, who enjoy sex enough not to mind if it becomes rote and boring. The subtle bids and requests for more variety can be passed aside because the sex "works." It can be easy not to take your partner's request seriously when you both orgasm most of the time. But even though this mundane path may be okay for a while, it may also lead to a partner looking elsewhere for more variety.

The most common predicament, in position #1, is people who want to please but don't know how. Having good sex takes more than just reading a Cosmo article at the dentist's office (although these can help!). It takes self-knowledge, opening your mouth to talk, perseverance and patience.

When to have logistical, specific talks to improve sex quality is a matter of debate even among professional sex therapists. You have to work out your own timing for discussing sexual scripts. How and whenever you do it, take your ideal sexual script (in writing) into the conversation. It will make everything very concrete. I have found that having this kind of conversation outside of the bedroom is good for more major issues, such as "I am feeling like sex is too much work lately" or "The same old, same old is boring me." But for small issues, such as exactly what spot to lick, you may find it better to talk during or right after sex while the spot is fresh in your mind.

Whatever route you choose (and even if you do both), take time to preplan the conversation to better explain what you need from each other.

Getting (and Giving) the Sex You Need

To gain clarity for yourself and your partner about what would make sex more fun for you, try some of these exercises. You will be surprised how arousing it can make you and your partner when you each think about, write down and talk about what you *really, really* want in your sex life.

Write Down Your Perfect Sexual Script— Both the Long and Short Version

Write down or type out *on paper* (so you both have a hard copy) how the flow of sex would go between you two in your perfect world. If you want to receive oral sex each time you make love, put it down. If you want a soft fingertip caressing along the sides of your breasts and then firm squeezing of the same—write it down. Sometimes sex is slow and relaxed. Sometimes it is a quickie. Write down your perfect version of both kinds. And don't be afraid to tell your partner when it is time to revamp a written sexual script because you are bored or waning in desire.

If you feel at a loss as to how to write down what you need, start by trying to mimic the following "Seven Stages of Foreplay." These are a kind of sexual baseline you can use to develop your own script.

Try Out the "Seven Stages of Foreplay"

I first heard Garrison Keillor use this phrase on National Public Radio while I was driving in the car and laughed out loud, then thought, "That about sums it up." The following sexual script is as good as any for creating satisfying lovemaking.

1) *Deep kissing*...enjoyed by almost everyone!

2) *Licking and nibbling* of necks, earlobes or other nonbreast and nongenital areas. Ladies, don't be too upset if he has none...other than the main event.

3) *Breast play.* Mix it up in terms of rough versus soft and sensual. And what feels good may change throughout her cycle each month.

4) *Oral sex on him.*

5) *Oral sex on her*....or "kill two birds with one stone" in the 69 position.

6) *Anal play* as deep or as fleeting as the players like, using fingers, tongues and/or toys.

7) *Intercourse.*

If you are looking to expand your sex life, working in these seven stages most times when you make love gives lots of time for experimenting and learning as well as for both partners to focus on what they like best. It doesn't need to take more than the average 15 minutes—but it can!

Focus on Your "Shiver Spots"

When you are writing down your ideal sexual script, think through the key words or locations that make you *shiver a bit* when you think about them. On me, there is a certain spot on my neck that if bitten correctly makes me shiver. For a guy, the shiver spot may be his wife licking and caressing his balls.

Underline these key words in your sexual script and share these with your partner. Memorize your partner's spots, say them aloud and *commit* yourself to them.

Straight Talk In and Out of the Bedroom

It is important to clearly hear one another's hints and act on them, even if the hints are nonverbal. This can mean hearing our DH say, "I haven't seen that hot pink lace thong for a while" and realizing it is time to wear it again. Guys, remember, many women prefer to guide their men with "MMMMmms" or "Oh that feels good" or lifting of the hips with a rhythmic thrusting toward our man during cunnilingus...these all say, "YES, KEEP DOING THAT!"

On the other hand, stillness and silence can (but don't always) mean "I am thinking about work" or "I wish you would stop doing that." If you are unsure what her silence meant during lovemaking, ask her. Ladies, moan, groan, give him a clue.

Try The Joy of Sex

When our lovemaking becomes too mechanical, Gil and I will start going through the pages of sex books like the latest edition of Dr. Alex Comfort's *The Joy of Sex*. One year we decided to try everything in the book in order (before Hollywood had the idea). This lasted for only 50 pages, but it was fun and took the thinking out of what to do each time. Now we enjoy Rinna & Kerner's *The Big, Fun, Sexy Sex Book*!

Keep it Fresh

Keep your body fresh. Make a commitment to keep unpleasant hygiene out of the way of good sex. Chronic bad breath, for instance, is often a sign of dental issues. Get a cleaning and checkup if your breath is a recurring comment from your partner! Brush your teeth before sex if it is "onion night" at dinner or almost every time, as we do, just because.

Take showers as needed before sex or clean your genitals by hand. My paradigm is "wash it up" (genitalia, that is) with a quick cleanup at the sink using the gentle, nonirritating Organix body wash and a warm washcloth.

Ladies, during oral sex men don't like encountering the bits of toilet paper or *smegma* (the white cheesy stuff from oils in your body) that accumulate in the folds of your labia. Feminine wipes aren't so good because they contain propylene glycol or glycerin and thus leave a funky over-sweet taste and can cause irritation. Washing your privates literally takes only two minutes. It can become part of your sexual script itself and keeps you from that awkward, "Don't go down there moment" which we save at our house for camping or spontaneous outdoor sex.

Guys, if you aren't circumcised, you can also develop smegma in the folds around your foreskin. Pull it back to wash under this area. But for all men, I guarantee that a fabulously clean cock will get more head!

For rimming or other anal play: frankly, guys, you grow more hair here than you know, and it can be hard to clean to the point that many women will want to lick or finger your anus. The easiest fix? Shave this area so that soap and water are simple to use for cleanup. A lightly flavored massage oil (e.g., Kama Sutra's Soaring Spirit) can make this part of your body more accessible and fun.

Pay Attention to Touch Type

The best way to know how to give a guy a good hand job is to watch him masturbate. Keep the lights low and *no* talking during this. Just watch what he does to pleasure himself. Notice where he is rough, where he is gentle and when he changes up the pattern.

Guys, the best way to know how to handle your lady's parts is not necessarily through watching her masturbate (although this can be fun) but rather by "partnered hand masturbation" in a few dedicated sessions during which you ask her to give you a number while you are touching her (1 to 5, with 5 awesome and 1 being ho-hum). Ask her to just whisper a number while you try this and that. Maybe a finger directly stroking the head of her clit is a "4" for a few seconds, but then it becomes a "1" because the sensitive tissue is getting overstimulated. Over a number of sessions, you'll be able to "hear" what she needs so that you can then practice these touch types. For more ways to improve your sensual touch check out the book *Red Hot Touch* by Jaiya and Hanauer.

One thing to keep in mind during sex is that men often don't realize how prone to irritation the head of the clitoris can get *before* a woman's orgasm. Guys, it is similar to *after* you have an intense orgasm and the tip of your cock is sensitive to touch—same thing, just at a different stage of the cycle...so please be gentle. She can always ask for harder!

Loving the Lube

Most women feel arousal-based sexual desire. After they are aroused then they feel the desire, which can be the opposite of men who feel desire and then become aroused. If sex is hurting (albeit without anyone meaning for it to) women are not going to feel aroused; unaroused, they won't feel desire; without desire, their lady parts never get wet. You can circumvent this issue by applying Pre-Seed inside the vagina before making love (while freshening up in the bathroom). This makes the foreplay wet and slippery, easier, more fun and leads to her feeling aroused, which fuels desire and triggers more of her own natural wetness most quickly. With the right lube in the right place, the tip of your cock or your finger (guys) can easily slide over her clit, teasing her. *If you try nothing else from this book, try applying Pre-Seed inside the vagina before starting foreplay and see what you think!* Many older women report to me that it has changed their lovemaking enjoyment!

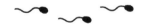

Give and Receive More Oral Sex

No place is sexual communication more needed than during oral sex. During penile-vaginal intercourse, we can use our bodies to guide rhythms and pressure. Oral sex is something the other partner "gives" to us. About 60% of married Americans give and receive oral sex, but many want to receive more than they are getting. Why aren't people bagging the oral sex they want? Usually this comes down to one of three things: a) a gross factor; b) an uncertainty factor; or c) selfishness.

Young people can be very self-centered in sex, especially guys. For me, a man's willingness to do "oral" and his enjoyment of the same has been a *required selection criterion* in my adult relationships. Ladies, whether you are 19 or 90, if you start having sex with a guy who can't be bothered to become intimate with your lady parts, show him the door. This is *not* what you want in a long-term relationship. Although cunnilingus may not be critical to you now, a man's disregard for worshiping your genital area (as he should) may not ever go away. Think twice before committing too much to a partner like this.

The gross-out factor is best dealt with by keeping yourself clean as we discussed (especially the grooves deep inside the vulva). It also may help if you shave, a lot. If you like cunnilingus but he doesn't like the hair, shave it every day or two in the shower...no big deal. Guys you can shave too. As mentioned, aging for men leads to increased hair growth along the shaft of your penis. This can be distracting during oral sex. We love and use the Venus® razors with the gel strips. They make it easy and nonirritating to quickly shave (on a daily basis) for partners who prefer this.

To get a man to enjoy cunnilingus if he's the type that is just put off by the whole thing, start initially with short sessions of light kisses and give him all the right audibles. Then as he relaxes each time you have sex, encourage him to stay a bit longer by praising him during the session with up and down hip movement and some "MMMMmms." Try putting a small pillow under your ass (to raise yourself up) and then bend your knees and bring your heels up toward your butt (as if in a yoga position). Open it all up to him—it is easier for him and allows him to better visualize what he is doing where and to correlate his moves with your reactions. It also makes you open and vulnerable to him at a time he may be feeling a bit intimidated. Dark or dim lighting is always a good equalizer for nervous folks too. And throughout the process, give praise!

For her on him, minimizing any gross-out of oral sex on men is of course linked to having a clean cock. Beyond that, if she feels choked because he is thrusting too deep, he may get less oral sex. And, of course, a huge concern for most gals is dealing with a mouthful of cum. It isn't always that fun to receive, and, men, if you have not ejaculated in a while, your wad will have a higher volume. Similarly, if you haven't drunk much water during the day, your ejaculate can be thick and highly concentrated with sugars (slimy sweet). This can turn off even the biggest fellatio fan.

Guys, as you ponder your sexual script, think about what aspect you like *most* in BJs. Having oral sex for arousal and foreplay is completely different than finishing sex with your cum in her mouth. Think about these two activities as separate events. Is your favorite part of a BJ the sensation of the arousal? If so, then use oral during the Seven Stages of Foreplay to get her giving you more that way; build it into your sexual script as part of normal foreplay. And guys, this is your time for the audibles...groan, moan, "Oh baby" it up so she knows you like it.

Ladies, focus on how soft and sensual his cock feels on the roof of your mouth; close your eyes and enjoy the sensation of it sliding in and out. Don't gag yourself unless, over time, you start to enjoy pushing the boundaries.

And remember, for women who don't like doing fellatio that much, not having it tied to ejaculation every time keeps her from being overwhelmed by it. It's better if she feels like she is an empowered tigress when she does it, so train her in the ways you need the oral sex without intimidating her. If coming in your lady's mouth is really all you want from oral sex, make sure to give her a rocking orgasm before you go there.

Overall, you can help your woman enjoy oral sex more by 1) staying hydrated so your semen is not too thick, 2) ejaculating frequently to reduce your semen volume, and 3) having a vasectomy when you are done with kids, again for less semen volume in her mouth.

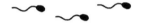

Discovering a new lover as adults was both scary and sexy for my new husband and I. Overall it made us more willing to bring the honesty that comes with age into our bedroom, sometimes with giggles, sometimes with disappointment and even sometimes with anger.

Chapter 13

Knights In Shining Armor & Dragon Slaying

In the late spring of 2003, Pre-Seed was flying out the door. And things couldn't have been more perfect for me! Gil and I were planning our summer wedding at a mountain lodge in north Idaho. We had already purchased 70 acres and had begun blending our five boys (ages six to eighteen) into a family (and an 1,800 sq ft manufactured home). I had just won the internationally renowned Young Andrologist Award—one of the highest achievements for someone in my field. Pre-Seed product sales and reviews were topping the charts. It was obvious to everyone involved with the company that Pre-Seed was going to be a game changer for trying-to-conceive couples. Additionally, BioOrigyn received an NIH Small Business Innovative Research grant to continue clinical studies on the arabinogalactan protection of sperm. It was looking like my "dream" spring!

During this time, we also hired new personnel for BioOrigyn including: a new board member who was a retired Johnson & Johnson manager eager to introduce Pre-Seed to the drugstore shelf, a new Chairman of the Board with substantial experience in biotechnology, and a proven CEO (also a woman) to lead us forward. These folks were looking to raise *real* money for a national Pre-Seed retail launch and for Bio to develop other AG-based fertility products. Best of all for me personally, I would be able to pare down my workload after Gil and I were married! We were ready for the big time.

But as so often happens when companies start to grow rapidly, the owners of Bio began to disagree on Pre-Seed's future direction. As we started drawing in out-of-town pharmaceutical expertise—with large investments planned through experienced biotechnology firms from Palo Alto, California—a battle ensued over who would control Bio's ownership during these changes: the founders or the venture capitalists. These power struggles culminated in an eventual shutdown of Bio shortly before my June wedding. It was stressful beyond words. I knew I could lose everything I had worked for over the past decade, including Pre-Seed. Initially I remained optimistic that the owners of Bio would work through our differences and agree to move forward in short order. Unfortunately, this was not to be the case. It would actually take months to resolve the issues and to reopen BioOrigyn. Luckily, I didn't know this at the time of my wedding celebration.

Dreams Come True

With the surreal company battle in the background, Gil and I married one another on a mountain meadow overlooking Lake Pend Oreille in Idaho. All five of our handsome sons—Casey, Ryan, Tyler, Rayne and Sayge—wore Western shirts, boots and cowboy hats. Despite the uncertainties and power struggles at work, this was one of the happiest days of my life. In our vows, I told Gil that going forward with him "I'd rather take ten seconds in the saddle than a lifetime of watching from the stands." These lyrics from rodeo star and singer Chris LeDoux expressed perfectly the wild bareback bronco ride of a life Gil and I were starting out with!

During the ceremony, the sun shone down on us and the smell of mountain spruce filled the air as friends and family sang together: "'Tis a gift to be simple, 'Tis a gift to be free; 'Tis a gift to come down where we ought to be" I knew I was where I "ought to be" next to Gil and our boys.

For a little while, I let go of the strife at the company and just loved the men in my life as we united our families into one. We were the "Rockin' JDK Ranch" short for "Joanna, Dennis and the Kids." On our farm in Eastern Washington, we weren't the Cliftons; we weren't the Ellingtons; we were a new blend of the two. Our boys rallied into our new family in a way that caused one of our ex's attorneys to refer to us as having "blended family nirvana." It wasn't perfect, of course, but from the beginning we shared those times of work, laughter and animal antics that country families are privileged to experience.

Power Struggles

But back at work the business conflicts awaited me. After a magical wedding and cozy honeymoon on the Oregon Coast, I returned to the heated negotiations of how to move Bio forward. As the owners of Pre-Seed stayed in a stalemate, supplies of the product began to dwindle. A November 2003 Seattle Post-Intelligencer news story explained the chaos this inventory shortage was causing in the TTC world as remaining boxes of Pre-Seed began to be sold by individuals on eBay. After the article's headline announcement, "Bidding is lively for sperm-friendly moisturizer," the story went on to inform the world that "A sperm-friendly moisturizer that helps women conceive is commanding sky high prices on eBay after the Spokane manufacturer ran out of supplies this summer." The article also reported that speculators on eBay were finding a market for Pre-Seed, "...selling it for three or four times its $19 retail price..."

Our distributor had told the PI, "Pre-Seed was immensely popular with women...It was definitely a star product for us... Apparently, the efficacy is amazing..." In fact, when Pre-Seed supplies ran out, this distributor "received complaints from customers who were upset that the product was no longer available." They even had to send a letter to their customers explaining that it wasn't their fault the Pre-Seed was out of stock.

The chat-rooms I had been part of, such as TCOYF, actually began linking women who needed product to women with unused *applicators* at home. In fact, one box of Pre-Seed was split between three couples...and resulted in three pregnancies!

From my side of things, the discouragement was beyond words as I watched people desperate for a product that could help them while, at the same time, I was powerless to move forward with the hopes and dreams we had held for the company just months before. I couldn't sleep at night and stopped eating...just as Gil and I were launching our new marriage.

Finally, in January of 2004, Gil and I, together with Gil's generous parents, were able to gain majority control of Bio and bring Pre-Seed back to market! Yet again another Seattle Post-Intelligencer article chronicled a portion of our journey. The January 5, 2004 headline informed readers that a "Former top exec of ING Fertility files suit" (remember ING Fertility was the lubricant division of BioOrigyn). The article explained how I "took the unusual legal action after the company's venture capitalists failed to respond to a settlement offer." The story further detailed how uncommon it was for entrepreneurs, such as myself, to file a lawsuit against their venture capital partners. One Seattle attorney quoted in the article stated that he had "never encountered a similar case in the Puget Sound region." Another quoted attorney explained, "Usually, what happens is that they [the founders and venture capitalists] work out a settlement..."

Chronicling an additional ordeal at the time, the article also reported that I had contacted the Spokane Police Department to request assistance with the recovery of $20,000 worth of Pre-Seed that I had suspected a former employee had stolen and was selling on eBay. This theft eventually did result in charges and partial restitution to Bio. Lastly, the reporter included a quote from me aptly summarizing my feelings on the 2003 business lessons I had learned: "I am pretty committed to not doing venture capital again. It about took my life's work. I don't want to do that again."

Pre-Seed Again

Finally, in December 2003, in spite of everything we had been through, we were almost ready to make Pre-Seed available again for TTC couples. As we waited for new product inventory to arrive, we began pre-order sales on the internet. This created a lot of excitement in trying-to-conceive chat-rooms as word spread that Pre-Seed was returning! In fact, in the last few weeks of the year we presold 1,500 units of Pre-Seed.

We also established new distribution channels with the top preconception websites of Fairhaven Health and Earth's Magic. These partners were so supportive of us and Pre-Seed that they agreed to pay us early for the product (before it shipped) so we could fund our employees' Christmas payroll.

Christmas break that year consisted of a "family project" with all the JDK Ranch boys folding white shipping boxes so we would be able to mail the Pre-Seed out as soon as it arrived. Every closet in the house was chock-full of these shipping boxes, all ready to go.

Finally the day came for our manufacturer to deliver the Pre-Seed by truck to the farm. Since regaining control of the company, we had figured that we would run the business out of a new warehouse on our farm. Construction of the facility was underway but not yet done when the product arrived. Instead, these initial orders of Pre-Seed would be sent out from our kitchen table where an assembly line had been set up waiting to process the ever growing stack of pre-orders. We were ready and waiting for product, with a system in place to dial in credit card numbers, type up labels and tape boxes shut. Our rural U.S. Post Office was about to get a large boost in activity!

On the day the product was to arrive from Idaho, there was a huge snowstorm with an eight-inch powder dump. I had to run to pick up the younger boys from school, and Gil was at his "real" job. The driver arrived carrying our Pre-Seed but couldn't navigate our farm's rather long, buried-in-snow driveway, so he had to leave the pallets of Pre-Seed wrapped in plastic on the side of the road. Our employee Julie, who was seven months pregnant, had gone to check in the product at the farm, but much to her surprise found the driver carefully unloading his pallets...along the road by our gate. With the snow continuing to fall, there was no time to lose getting the Pre-Seed into the house! So Julie and our second son, Ryan, started transferring cases of Pre-Seed from the pallets through the deep snow, load by load, into her ISUZU® Trooper to transport them the quarter mile up to our house. By the time the rest of us converged on the farm, all the newly manufactured Pre-Seed was safely stacked in our family room, waiting for the assembly line processing to begin. I am sad there is no picture of a very pregnant Julie trudging through calf-deep snow to bring Pre-Seed back to the TTC couples of the world!

For the next two days we had a major Pre-Seed work "party," processing orders to get them out the door. Our oldest son, Casey, was hunched over the dial-up credit card machine (which at the farm was extremely slow) for 16 hours both days. The rest of us had raw fingers from folding packing slips and taping boxes shut. Thank heavens the kids had pre-folded all the shipping boxes over

Christmas break. I always felt like the people who received these "home-packed" boxes of Pre-Seed in January 2004 received a special JDK Ranch blessing!

After we started up Pre-Seed sales again, things changed quickly for our company and for Gil and me personally. He soon stopped working as a professor at WSU so that he could work for the company full time and oversee Bio's manufacturing and clinical research. With this we went from loving each other and seeing each other a few hours a day to loving each other and working together all day, every day. That was a lot of togetherness!

Sex and Stress or Sex as Stress

It goes without saying that Gil and I started our marriage under intense emotional stress. Five kids are a lot more than two or three (as I or he had respectively). But most of our stress involved the battle for control of BioOrigyn. The stakes were very high with the potential loss of my past decade of work, as well as possible legal risks. And these battles were personally very expensive, with attorneys hired on several different fronts.

As we entered into a new work relationship together, we experienced new layers of power struggles. Before, we had both been "the boss" in our own realms. Now we knew we needed to stay focused on our sex life if our marriage was to last, even during those times that we butted heads at work or at home. This knowledge grew not just from our own lives but also from the many couples I had heard from and worked with over the years. I also knew that research is clear about sex in the first years of a marriage: if a couple can learn to have good sex together that first year or so, the couple's chance of staying together remains higher than for those couples who have unsatisfying sex during this life phase. We were also old enough to know that sometimes sex can get boring, in the day in and day out of life. And boring sex can put partners at risk for finding excitement outside of each other.

Research has shown that, biologically, a woman's sexual attraction to her partner can start to lessen within the first year of a relationship due to that ancient mating strategy of sexual selection. Her sexual desire can drop off as her DNA tells her it is time to go find the dominant male again that can help make those genetically supercharged babies. Men often notice this happening in the woman. When they see this decline in her "horniness," they often interpret it as a betrayal (a "bait and switch" by the gals—"she got me into this relationship with lots of sex, but now that I'm in, she's not nearly as interested in it."). But, guys please don't forget the probable *biological* reason for this change and stay committed to making sex work for this gal. Your commitment to your intimacy together can help her forget her sexual blaahs and become even more bonded to you. And ladies, look carefully at your own motivations. If this is the man you want to stay with for many years, understand your DNA's pull and override it by making sex so fun that *you* can't resist it either!

Radical Center Ruminations - Overshadowed by the media attention on the misogyny and sexual violence against women in our culture is the "Catch-22" that the "nice" guy has during sex. Rape is obviously not okay, but if we consistently tell our young men they have to "ask" before making any advance in sexual touching, they may just decide that the most respectful way to approach intimacy is to hang back and let the woman craft the sexual script. This would be a bio-sexual mistake, in many cases, as you can learn at the "girl's" table at Starbucks by listening to the complaining (especially among more educated women with equally educated male partners). Many of these women feel that their guys are so passive and undemanding in bed that they (the gals) end up bored to tears.

Cultural sexual scripts, dictated by certain puritanical or rigidly feminist women, demand that men leave their aggression and intensity outside the bedroom door; these scripts are no less detrimental to society, in my science-based view, than are cultural scripts of women as physical objects. In the end, emasculating men during sex will not fulfill women; women will end up dumping the "nice" guy for the jerky alpha male who may not be able to distinguish between being a stud in the sack and being too aggressive or, even, violent. For a fun primer on more Tarzan in the bedroom, check out Eve Kingsley's book *Just Fuck Me! - What Women Want Men to Know About Taking Control in the Bedroom (A Guide for Couples)*.

Sex Tips for the Sexually Committed

Sex within a committed relationship can be exciting and sustaining. But these relationships that get us through the highs and lows of everyday life also need a commitment to good sex. It isn't a one-way street. Here are some lessons learned from real life and from sexual science for making commitment much more fun.

Schedule Ahead

Even when you are trying to honor each other, it is easy to miss each other's cues. It is wise to map out a plan together for when to have sex for the week or at least over the next few days. Your partner can then make sure s/he isn't running an errand or making a business call while you're waiting back home in bed. Many of the most wonderful things in life are preplanned and scheduled—sex can be one of these, especially if you have children and/or both work. For most of us, scheduling sex is not a show of weakness in the relationship but, instead, evidence of our sexual and romantic health. If it happens additionally outside of the schedule—yippee!—but knowing it is on the calendar can help you both relax about the topic.

Don't Wait

If you start kissing and thinking "should we"...you should! Haven't we all postponed until later, only to fall exhausted into bed that night, sexless. Usually there really is time. Let the kids think you are taking a shower or tell the boss traffic was bad. This is maintenance for the love you share with a life partner. This is important stuff! It only takes fifteen minutes or so. Just do it. Sex releases the hormones you need to enjoy each other and stay in partnership. If you are a woman for whom vaginal sex takes a while, get a vibrator to use with him for these "quickies." He will most likely find the addition of this new toy quite fascinating!

Make Sex a Priority

Life is busy. If you don't prioritize sex, life will bump it way down on the list. Here are some simple ways to make sex a priority.

Get the TV out of the bedroom! Intimacy and TV do not go together (short of watching erotic films together occasionally). If you value your relationship, keep sex a priority and move the TV to another room. Even if you are scared to death to try this—do it for two weeks and see how it goes! Or, cover the box with a beautiful blanket and pretend it isn't there. If you are highly TV-addicted, try a joint custody arrangement. One week the TV works in the bedroom, one week it is "broken."

Don't rely only on waiting to have sex as the last thing at night. Find ways not to just have sex at the end of the day when our bodies are tired and slow to respond. One of the reasons sexual affairs are so novel and fun for people is that they often occur in the middle of the day. So schedule a "doctor's appointment" once a quarter or miss work occasionally to have a tryst with your spouse. Rent a hotel at five p.m. near your work on your anniversary. Even if you have to pay for the room for the night, a good hour of wild afternoon sex will make you feel pampered and naughty. Trust me—it is well worth it.

Have sex before you go out to dinner. On date nights, switch things up and make love *before* dinner. Libido can tank on a full stomach and after a few glasses of wine. Enjoy each other sexually and *then* go out—this allows dinner in the "afterglow" without having to worry about being too tired or having too much to drink. To better understand the negative impacts of drinking on sexual performance, check out Dr. Castellanos' *Is Alcohol to Blame for Delayed Ejaculation* at *thesexmd.com* (the short answer... yes!).

Disconnect the telephone line. Unplug answering machines, turn off phones...make sure distractions don't interrupt you. Nothing can tank intimacy like hearing your mom's voice during foreplay or receiving a steady stream of text pings! Work and family can wait— remember this is all about *prioritizing **making** love*.

Make Love Not War

Many couples fight over "little things" either because of unresolved sexual tension or in a way that having sex can resolve. Gil and I try to make love every couple days. Sometimes if we don't, we get snarly with each other. In the past this would escalate into full-scale fights, hurt feelings and no sex (hit rewind and repeat). Now we try to get to the sex part even if we are still mad at each other. This way we are dispersing any of the negativity associated with built-up sexual tension and saving the fighting for more serious issues (like the laundry).

Schedule Gourmet Sex

Maintenance sex is great—it works well; you know the buttons to push and the moves to make to find fulfillment for both of you—but it often happens in a time bind between activities and the bedtime clock. So, every few months at least, schedule a night of *Gourmet Sex* with the some of the moves we have discussed previously.

Also bring in the massage oils and candles...take your time. Try the new positions and focus on conveying how much you love your spouse as you please him or her. Talk ahead of time (if you wish) about the new things you want to try out. Then try them out in this unrushed setting. Even if things don't work out exactly as you hoped, you will still feel cherished. Tomorrow, the old Route 66 will still be there if needed, but for today, the fine wine is tasted and enjoyed.

Be a Bit Naughty

We all have sexual fantasies—we let them fill our minds in order to amp up our arousal now and then. BDSM images can help us in this regard. BDSM (Bondage, Discipline, Sexual Sadism and Masochism) is sex using physical restriction, role-playing scenarios, exchanging who has the power and types of contact that cause pain. A wide range of people report engaging in varying forms of BDSM or "kink"— most common are biting each other, tying each other up, spanking and acting out fantasies. Numbers range from 2% of the population identifying themselves as practitioners of kink to 36% of Americans saying they have used blindfolds or bondage at some time in their love lives, and over 50% who have bitten a partner.

In reality, BDSM behaviors fall on a continuum from mild to extreme. Rather than pain being at the core of BDSM, it is more about using exchanges of power in an erotic context to increase sexual pleasure. One person takes control of the sexual setting to dominate the sexual script while the other person is submissive to this script. The overarching BDSM credo is "safe, sane, and consensual." While in the past BDSM was stigmatized medically as sexual deviation, kink practitioners are no more likely to be psychologically distressed or sexually dysfunctional than the general population. In fact, in studies these folks exhibit *higher* levels of subjective wellbeing than nonkink users. Not surprisingly, they report greater psychological health and better use of language to explicitly communicate their sexual desires to a partner than do nonBDSM lovers.

Can you have a great sex life without ever using a single BDSM technique? Sure you can. But if you are trying to keep a great sex life through turmoil and/or boredom, and you feel "stuck" as to what to do, think about trying some BDSM sex, even in its mildest forms. You might find a whole new world of sexual health open up in you and your marriage.

Like many American women, I have a *Fifty Shades of Grey* story. In my own version of the Amazon advertisement where the woman is trying to hide her Fifty Shades book from her family, I devoured the first book. Sneakily, I hid it in a magazine while reading it under a tree with hundreds of high school students and their parents around me at a weekend Cross Country meet. The next week, DH got a lot of sex, including spanking and tying each other up with a soft nylon rope brought up from the barn. We had kind of "forgotten" about this kind of fun since we had changed to a new bed without a frame. Plus we were in a mundane spot, where sex had gotten boring and our effort to improve it minimal. After I shared a few *Fifty Shades* pages with him, DH got creative and ran one long rope all the way under the bed so that it came out on either side, and we could use it to tie each other up.

This diversion into light BDSM was just what we needed to start having more fun with sex. We both laughed during lovemaking for the first time in a long time, and it reminded us that we could spend time trying new things and didn't need to be so "goal" oriented to get to orgasm. The rope was all fun and good until we shampooed the carpet and forgot it was there…a bit awkward when the boys helped us move our bed later that month!

Several research papers, as well as many other voices (e.g., at *BlogHer.com*), question if *Fifty Shades of Grey* is really about BDSM or just another take on the romance novel with an extreme dominant male using BDSM props. Although Anastasia is depicted as finding pleasure during most of the couple's sexual interactions, she is simultaneously terrified that she will be physically and emotionally hurt and yearns for a "normal" relationship with Christian. The story line is the quintessential Adversary Transformation tale. It is interesting to note that the many readers of this book have not continued to read other BDSM genre novels, instead they have returned to their usual romance novels. My vote: Fifty Shades was an awesome romance novel with lots of arousing language to make everyone who read it or who partnered with someone who read it happy!

Radical Center Ruminations - One cautionary note from my review of the science on BDSM: the highest percentage of participation for women in kink is between the ages of 16 and 19. Are these young women participating in BDSM for pleasure or to please? Is kink sexually satisfying, or are they just performing compliant sex with a new twist?

Given that three quarters of the Submissives in BDSM are women and men are six times more likely to be the Dominant, I find suspect the statements that most BDSM is about "increasing sexual pleasure" for both participants versus just more enactment of our mating strategies with the dominant male and ritual female submission (albeit with a modern veneer of cool). I hope all these young women are having their minds blown by great sex in these situations, but anything that is supposed to be reciprocal with this much of a gender skew is a red flag to me.

Even though Gil and I worked diligently at prioritizing sex in our new marriage, with the stresses of a growing family and the Pre-Seed business turn-around, we were unprepared for our next hurdle. At 43 I began to have extremely disruptive premenopausal symptoms, but due to their earlier than usual onset, I was unaware of their cause. These "mystery" symptoms and a subsequent five-year stint of surgeries and medical complications were about to challenge our commitment to sex and intimacy in a profound and prolonged manner.

Chapter 14

Sometimes You're Up – Sometimes You're Down

W hen it comes to my own reproductive physiology, I can sometimes be a bit slow to catch on (like not understanding how I had gotten pregnant in 1992). It would take me over five years and a lot more suffering to finally figure out what was "wrong" with me during this phase of my life. During this time I also learned that everything that was happening to me was completely normal physiology for someone in *perimenopause*. Part of my confusion was that I would visit physicians and be told, "It's just stress. You still have your period. Your symptoms aren't from menopause yet." Misinformation such as this did nothing to help me solve the mystery of my ever-changing physical and mental health status in my 40s.

What Is "Menopause"?

Since I was somewhat clueless about menopause in spite of all my training, let me quickly review with you what the term means. In actuality, there are three stages to this life-changing event. These consist of pre (before), peri (during) and post (after) *menopause* (i.e., when menstruation stops). We often refer to women in the later part of their life as "menopausal women," but these women are actually postmenopausal.

During puberty in teenage girls, the changing hormones and emotional roller coaster take about a year or two to get through. In contrast, "the change" as menopause is affectionately (or not) referred to can take many *years*. When I married Gil, I was entering the premenopause zone. Going through this phase lasts between four to eight years for most women. The average age of a woman's final period (her menopause) is 51. This of course makes our 40s—and into our 50s—a wild, hormonal ride. As our bodies *slowly* bring ovulation to a halt, the sex steroids in our bloodstream begin to swing wildly between high and low levels. The communication systems between our brain and ovaries that once confined these hormones to neat monthly waves resulting in the cycles of ovulation followed by our period (unless we became pregnant) become completely disengaged and dysfunctional. Our bodies make up for this lack of productive dialogue between the brain and ovaries by taking turns shouting at or ignoring each other (hormonally speaking). The result is erratic swings in estrogen levels and declining testosterone during these menopausal changes. *One-time* measurement of blood hormones during this time to diagnose if health problems are menopause-related may not be very helpful. This is because it isn't the absolute hormone levels that cause the symptoms but rather the *changing* levels, just as we saw for women with postpartum depression.

Adding insult to injury, during the menopause transition, the receptors that bind to the sex steroids in our bodies often stop working correctly, so our cells can't even register the hormones that are present.

Symptoms of "The Change"

In spite of my PhD in reproductive physiology, in my 40s I had no idea I was suffering from many common premenopausal symptoms.

While some were annoying, others represented significant health risks and dramatically decreased my overall quality of life and my functioning at home and at work. I hope you will learn from my mistakes.

Before we take a look at my individual story, let's review the symptoms that suggest a woman is beginning her menopausal journey, even if she still is having her period.

- Fatigue (increased in severity and frequency)

- Urologic symptoms (increased urge to pee and leaking urine)

- Weight redistribution to the abdomen

- Recurrent urinary tract infections

- Sexual dysfunction (dryness, loss of libido, poor orgasm ability)

- Depression

- Anxiety

- Severe mood swings

- Cognitive symptoms (word failure and memory difficulty)

- Vasomotor symptoms—hot flashes, night sweats, rapid or racing heart rate

- Sleep disturbances—can't fall asleep, can't stay asleep

- Pain syndromes (decreased pain tolerance, increased nerve and muscle pain)

- Headaches

- Dry, itchy skin patches

- GI symptoms (diarrhea or constipation)

- Autoimmune diseases (rheumatoid, lupus, psoriatic arthritis)

If you have several of these symptoms, find a physician who specializes in menopause and aging in women as proven by the provider's membership in menopause medicine or aging medicine societies. You deserve a well researched and thought out plan for this new phase of life, *not just a prescription for antidepressants and sleeping pills*. But please know you will need to do some research on your own. With your menopausal "car" veering off course, you can't just "hand the keys" to your doctor.

Each woman is unique and each has her own life goals during menopause. If you decide to join the Shaker religion and commit to a lifetime of prayer and celibacy, your handling of menopause will likely be different from that of the triathlete woman with a super sexy husband who wants to enjoy an active intimate life into her 90s. Most of us are somewhere in between these extremes, but several things are critical to remember for all of us. First, there is no doctor on the planet to whom your menopause decisions are more critical than they are and will be to you. No one else can or should make a decision *for* you during the menopause change. These decisions will likely impact HALF of your life, so it is better to choose protocols that keep your options open. Your life now won't always be the life you are living. Many women who go through divorce in their forties or fifties can't imagine they will ever be with a partner again. Statistics say you will, so don't make decisions that involve swearing off sex and men (or women) lightly. I am approached all the time by women in their 70s and 80s who wish they had started or stayed on hormones but can't go back in time (based on our current medical recommendations).

One of the best lay reviews for the symptoms of early menopause is Suzanne Somers' *I'm Too Young for This!* This book just came out. I wish I had had such a great resource when I was in my mid forties. It would have helped me find solutions for my physical problems and "mood disorders" much sooner. And I would have realized that I was not alone or even unique in my hormonal chaos.

Have I Lost My Mind?

Premenopause for me started with patches of extremely itchy skin on my arms. (I had to laugh that Suzanne's book on her early menopause symptoms starts off with a chapter "It Started with an Itch"!) Over the following months I graduated to hot flashes during the day and night sweats in bed. At the time, I thought they were just symptoms from all the stress at work. These physical changes are called "vasomotor" symptoms of menopause. The most disruptive was when I began to develop sporadic blushing. For seemingly no reason at all, I would start to blush across my chest and face. It mortified me and also made the people I was talking to uncomfortable. The blushing happened so frequently I became afraid of meeting with people professionally and took to wearing turtlenecks so that it wouldn't show.

Eventually I began having debilitating anxiety attacks, something I had never experienced before. Usually these were triggered while standing in line, such as at the checkout counter of the grocery store. We had four teenage boys in our house back then, and I would routinely fill a grocery cart to overflowing. But the panic attacks would cause me to abandon my full cart at the store as I rushed outside to get some air and drive home empty-handed. I was starting to worry that maybe I was developing true mental health issues.

Over the next five years I would also be evaluated for Celiac disease for intermittent GI problems, be admitted to the emergency room twice for a racing heart, and eventually develop an autoimmune disease. My body had read the above menopausal symptom list, even if I hadn't!

As my anxiety got worse, I became very self-conscious of the aging changes and weight gain in my upper arms, abdomen and face. I felt like if I ran into someone I hadn't seen in a while, they would think, "Do I know her?" So I started staying more on the farm and would wear a hat and sunglasses if I went out. Looking back, I am amazed at how profound these changes were, but also how incremental so that neither hubby nor I sat up and took notice that I was headed on the path to becoming a "crazy old lady." At one point we discussed whether I needed antidepressants, but I knew I wouldn't take them as I didn't want to mess up my decreasing libido. Of course I didn't realize at the time that all of the above symptoms are commonly a part of pre and perimenopausal physiology as our sex steroid levels change and our brain chemistry becomes disrupted.

Menopause, a True Mind F...

Menopause causes dramatic alterations in the serotonin chemistry of our brain. Most of us understand that the chemical serotonin helps protect us from mood disorders, but it also does much more than that. Nearly all of our approximately 40 million brain cells are influenced by serotonin in some manner. Serotonin impacts mood, sexual function, appetite, sleep, memory, temperature regulation and social behavior. Hmmm...all the things that menopause messes with! That is because during menopause the changing estrogen levels cause our serotonin-sensitive neurons in the brain to begin dying, starting with the cells that control our emotions, then those involved in thinking (cognition) and finally those of our physical function. Depression and anxiety are often some of the first symptoms of approaching menopause. The more widely a woman's hormones fluctuate during this time, the greater her risk of developing depression. Often this can occur in women with no previous history of depression or anxiety.

The risk of developing mood disorders is *most prominent* in women with other body (vasomotor) changes, such as hot flashes, night sweats, sleep disorders or a racing heart (like I had); therefore, ladies, don't just think of hot flashes as "an inconvenience." They can be a sign that your estrogen levels are changing dramatically and act as a signal to you to watch for depression or anxiety.

To deal with the mood disorders of menopause, almost **25%** of American women 40 to 59 are on selective serotonin reuptake inhibitors (SSRI) antidepressants—this is an unbelievably high percentage of women! And remember—SSRIs have a *dramatically negative impact on libido, sexual desire and sexual function*. So just as a woman's body is going through the loss of the hormones that provide for her female sexual desire and arousal, one in four of us are also taking medications that in and of themselves cause a significant decrease in sexual desire and arousal. Now folks, that is crazy!

Disappointingly, many women (and even some doctors) don't realize that taking hormone replacement therapy (HRT) to resupply estrogen and testosterone may reverse these aging changes in the brain that lead to depression and/or anxiety. Several studies have found that some women do not even need the antidepressants once they start HRT. Women who have hot flashes with concurrent depression especially experience a strong psychological benefit from estrogen patch therapy, even without added antidepressants. For example, in one study 68% of women on estrogen therapy *alone* had full remission of depression symptoms compared to 20% in the placebo group (no medications).

For the anxiety aspect of menopause, *testosterone* has been shown in placebo-controlled studies to be the most effective sex steroid. Specifically, women on testosterone have a greater sense of wellbeing, significantly greater improvements in mood and decreases in anxiety as compared to women who did not take testosterone replacement.

It makes physiologic sense for menopausal women with mood disorders (where medically appropriate) to at least try hormone replacement since it can protect the serotonin sensitive cells in the brain, improving depression and anxiety while also enhancing sexual function, versus just using SSRI antidepressants that can further *damage* sexual function. Make sure your doctor has you on the latest methods for dealing with depression and anxiety during menopause. It can mean the difference between keeping sex alive at your house or not.

Radical Center Ruminations – The use of hormone replacement, such as in the form of estrogen patches, the Mirena® IUD and testosterone gels, is being increasingly recommended for women with depression during times of hormone fluctuations, such as during premenstrual syndrome, postpartum depression and perimenopausal depression. On the other hand, several studies have shown that the use of antidepressants during these times may be counterproductive in some women. Recent authors worry that a subset of women with severe premenstrual syndrome or perimenopausal depression (caused by hormone changes) are being misdiagnosed as bipolar and "inappropriately" placed on psychopharmacology drugs. In contrast, using hormone therapy to stabilize sex steroid blood levels may better help these women. In a 2014 published scientific commentary, J. Studd writes, "The hormonal causation of certain common types of depression in women and the successful treatment by estrogens should be understood by psychiatrists and gynecologists." Sadly, they are not. And because the response of a woman to sex steroid changes is often inherited, severe depression during these times should also be openly discussed within families and with each woman's health provider.

Even while I was struggling through these hormone horrors, Pre-Seed and our company continued to thrive. Independent clinical studies from renowned experts, such as Dr. Ashok Agarwal at the Cleveland Clinic Foundation, showed Pre-Seed's safety for sperm and its efficacy for use by couples who were trying to conceive. Pre-Seed also gained the *first-ever* clearance ("approval") by the FDA of any product as a fertility lubricant that was safe to use when couples were trying to conceive.

Then, in 2007, CVS pharmacy® (CVS) asked to carry Pre-Seed in its national sales line (CVS has about 7,500 stores in the U.S.). CVS is often an early adopter of new technology so we weren't surprised that they were the first chain to consider Pre-Seed. When a product gets to the national shelf of major chains, like CVS, it is critical that sales meet or exceed expectations and that inventory supplies not run out. Failure to accomplish these two goals will lead the product on a rapid trip to the clearance cart and removal from shelves. After a great deal of consideration, Bio asked CVS to wait a bit longer until we felt fully ready for the commitment to both the increased inventory and the ramped up marketing required to support this move. Our forecasts suggested this would take us a year, maybe less. Little did we know that, yet again, we were in for a rough ride before we would be able to reach this step.

To Hell in a Hand Basket

One January morning in 2008 after I had driven the boys to school, I trotted over some ice near our front door and my foot went out from underneath me. I crumpled to the ground screaming in pain. Gil came running out of the house and after one glance refused to let me look down at my leg because it was so badly broken and displaced. He loaded me into our Chevy Suburban and rushed me to the nearest ER. Within hours I was in surgery being operated on by a physician who was headed to Hawaii in two days and had been up all weekend on an emergency call. As I was coming out of anesthesia, I was screaming in pain. I knew something was horribly wrong and was very concerned about having a cast around my ankle. Given my level of pain, I was pretty sure I had compartment syndrome in which the blood supply to the nerve is cut off as the tissues swell with nowhere to expand to because of the rigid cast. I had seen horses coming out of surgery with this condition. They will literally beat themselves to death with the cast if it is not removed. The nurses and physician, however, kept telling me my pain was normal. I took pain pills, and Gil took me home. At home, I studied my cast and realized I needed to take it off before even more damage occurred. Unfortunately, I removed the cast too late. The nerve was already compromised and the constant resulting nerve pain, which I described to my doctor as "worse than childbirth," would trigger a whole cascade of health complications over the next five years. During the following months, I had to have several more surgeries on the ankle and ended up with an infection of the bone plate. I lived on crutches for seven months, and the nerve pain continued day and night...never changing, never lessening. In a stroke of even worse luck, I broke a toe on my good leg, tripping over my crutches as I hobbled around! Then I couldn't even walk at all for several weeks.

When it rains, it pours. The day after my last ankle surgery in May of the "bad year," I was lying on the couch reading a book. Gil and our son Ryan were on a horseback ride. Moments later I heard yelling and saw Ryan running to the house. "Joe, Dad came off Sonny [his horse] and hit a tree!" At a gallop, his horse had cut right on some trails while Gil kept going straight, straight into a two-foot wide pine tree. We got the Suburban (which was getting a lot of medical use lately) and drove out into the woods where Gil lay on the ground. The tree had just missed his head (no helmet) and fractured his pelvis into seven pieces. The long and the short of this— now we were both on crutches! I had been on them so long that some people thought Gil was using them in some weird sympathy stunt.

Throughout all these months, we were glad we knew something about the importance of sex and how to keep it going, but of course, as you can imagine, our intimacy was at times a bit comic. We would have to move very gingerly around each other, with lots of grunting and groaning and experimenting on what did and did not work. The Seven Stages of Foreplay were no longer possible because of positioning issues. We emphasized functional sex to find as easily and quickly as possible some release and pain mediation.

The icing on the cake of this bad karma year was when Gil and I discovered that a company we had once considered for our manufacturing had begun selling a knock off Pre-Seed product— including using a scientific illustration at their product website that Gil had created for marketing Pre-Seed. Bio filed federal infringement and false advertising claims against this product. Over the next eight months, Gil and I put everything we had into this battle. We withdrew funds from our retirement accounts and sold a car. We stopped paying ourselves and cut back on all nonessential Bio expenses. Sadly, we knew that yet again we wouldn't be ready for national stores for a while.

In the end, we "resolved" the litigation. The knock off would no longer be sold in the U.S., and Bio now owned the rights to the knock off product's name! But the physical and emotional stress of this year took its toll.

One day during the lawsuit, our attorneys videotaped me for a practice run through on my testimony. I was horrified when I saw the tape. I looked fat and old; in fact, I was unrecognizable to myself. I started crying in dismay. Our attorney told Gil to make an emergency run to Nordstrom with me to find something attractive to wear for the courtroom (gotta love the lady lawyers!). I had to find something with a turtleneck (for the blushing), something that would cover up my belly fat and something that wouldn't trigger hot flashes (sleeveless). This was *not* a fun shopping trip. After more tears, we left with two outfits I could wear.

At the end of this year, I almost let my perimenopausal body image stress and my overall anxiety keep me from an amazing professional opportunity. I was contacted by National Geographic to see if I could help make a documentary about sperm transport through the woman's body. I initially told them "no" because I felt so insecure about how I would look on camera. Thankfully, Gil would not let me refuse to do the film. He reminded me that I had important information for people and that I *enjoyed* teaching human sexuality. Together, we went to Toronto for several days of photo shoots for *The Great Sperm Race* (also aired as *Sizing Up Sperm* in some locations). I had to wear tennis shoes the whole shoot (as I always did back then because of my ankle) which didn't make me feel very chic. I also told the entire film crew (ten young, "hip" guys and Jennifer Beamish, a fabulous producer) that I *would* be having hot flashes and they *would* need to stop shooting for me when this happened, which they of course agreed to. Four times that day, we had to stop everything as this group of 20 to 30 year-old guys gathered around me waving folders and magazines to try to cool me down! They were awesome. I also ended up riding a bike in one scene—for the first time since my ankle fracture. Although a bit wobbly at first, it was just like, well, just like riding a bike!

Actually, I loved doing the film. People all over the world still email me to say they have recently seen the show. In fact, my nephew who attends a very conservative boarding school in the jungles of India told me his Sex Ed class showed the movie this year. Needless to say, he was shocked to see "Auntie Joe" in the film! But it helped me realize that even when I thought I wasn't functioning very well during this dark time, I was still creating information of lasting value for others by sharing my research and life's work.

I am not sure I would have been able to do the film without the support structure at home. Luckily, our oldest son Casey was back at the farm for a stint and kept the animals fed when Gil and I were on crutches (with help in the evenings from the other boys). Later that year, Gil stood by me at every moment during the documentary taping. He helped push me through my body image insecurity, my physical pain and my fear of riding a bike again. From all this I learned one of the great truths of menopause—don't blame your spouse! He is generally trying his best to serve you through one of your toughest times in life, when all the systems in your body are changing as we humans now live beyond our reproductive lifespan. This second half of life that we all take for granted today never existed for the vast majority of our ancestors! We are just learning how to navigate these years, complete with excitement, fulfillment and sometimes frustration.

Changing Bodies, Changing Selves

During our first decade of marriage, Gil and I had many circumstances that negatively impacted our intimacy and called for adjustments to keep sex fulfilling. From job stress, to hormone changes, to chronic pain and health problems, many outside issues could have shut down our lovemaking if we had let them. Small things began to more easily get in the way of good sex as we continued aging. What once would have been ignored (a phone ringing, the dog barking, garlic breath) could now destroy the mood. Around the time of the National Geographic shoot, I recall "the not-so-great sex year." We fought more about sex than any other topic during this time. I think it could have undone our relationship, especially if either of us had had someone else barking up our tree (providing emotional support and fun that could have lured us into an affair).

This year started innocently enough. Gil had some dental repairs done on his front teeth that changed the size and shape of his teeth. Around this same time I, as a middle-aged woman, wanted fuller lips and had my first JUVÉDERM® lip injections done. Who would have known that this would so negatively impact our sex lives? Now, my thicker lips started contacting Gil's new teeth when we kissed. Not only did this hurt, it also made me sad because kissing him now was so different than it had been before. I would make suggestions on how to make the kissing better, or sometimes get angered by it. Soon kissing became a loaded event in our lives. We would both get frustrated and feel like the other person wasn't trying to make it work. This would then carry forward into our sex lives. Sometimes our parts stopped working and there were no successful orgasms to be had, making us even more frustrated and angry.

We started out responding to the "kissing" situation as if it were isolated. We didn't yet realize that if we had viewed our intimacy as a living being, we would have seen that it was under attack on several fronts. My menopausal body changes, his aging changes, and the kissing issue were all weakening the health and condition of our lovemaking.

For instance, because of my approaching menopause, my genital tissues were thinning. Thus, the lining of my vulva and clitoris became more sensitive and easily irritated. Lovemaking, as we had done it for years, now sometimes left me feeling sore and overstimulated across the head of my clitoris. Even though I would still regularly orgasm, sex would leave me irritated over my clitoris, triggering negative flashbacks of the provoked vestibulodynia I had experienced in my 20s. At first I tried to ignore the fact that our foreplay was irritating me instead of turning me on. I decided, "Well, if I can just get to my orgasm, we'll be okay." But over time it got worse, so finally I tried to explain to Gil what wasn't working during sex.

After all the fighting about the kissing, he heard my new requests to "work" on the quality of our sex as criticism (okay...to be fair, they were often such). These discussions even sometimes ended our sex before it really got going. To make matters worse, what would feel good for me one day wouldn't feel so good the next. I felt truly clueless as to how to explain what I needed beyond just saying, "I need better sex!" My attempts to explain what was or was not working during intercourse were *not* a turn on for hubby who was headed into his 50s as well.

There were no good guys or bad guys here. But as is commonly reported in research, my decreased sexual fulfillment was leading to hubby's own lack of sexual enjoyment too. Since without his "participation" things couldn't happen, we decided to have him start taking Viagra® so that missteps or miscommunications wouldn't end the night so suddenly. I also got a book for us to read that I saw at a local bookstore called *She Comes First* by Ian Kerner about oral sex techniques. It seemed surreal to us that after years of successful marriage and sex together that, in our 50s, two smart scientists had to start over in learning how to please each other.

But we pressed on. We read together, looking at diagrams in the book, and practiced a few "dry runs" which weren't sex but just "Is this what he means?" exercises. We *loved* the Viagra® that allowed us to keep things going through thick and thin. And through it all, Pre-Seed inserted vaginally as I washed up for sex helped us immensely, keeping things feeling wet and sexy. Applying 1 gram of Pre-Seed deep inside as part of my pre-sex routine worked much better as I got older rather than stopping intercourse to use the lubricant *if* we needed it.

Although things got better, I could tell that I would need to do something differently if I was going to maintain my sexual health into the second half of my life. I was no longer unclear on whether or not I would do HRT after menopause. I loved having intense orgasms and enjoyed sex way too much to give those up mid-way on my journey through life. For me, it just became a matter of time until I would start on sex steroid supplementation through hormone replacement. Although I remained confused on exactly what kind of hormone replacement I would use, I knew I didn't want to lose my libido and desire for sex.

When Sex is Just a Headache

Sex without pleasure is messy, uncomfortable and quite frankly boring. Why bother? Because if you are in a partnership, it is important to remember that the sexual science is very clear. Where sex goes, so goes love. This is no exaggeration. Also, sex is good exercise and helps release tension and stress to improve your mood and outlook. Over many studies looking at numerous outcomes, good sex helps maintain a person's quality of life. Even if we are just having it with ourselves.

In spite of this, *hypoactive sexual desire disorder* (HSDD), or low sex drive, is the most common sexual complaint among women, constituting nearly half of all cases of people seeking clinical assistance for sexual dysfunction. Because we know that sexual satisfaction is part of relationship satisfaction, most of us realize that to be in a marriage we not only need to have sex but also should *want* to have sex. In spite of this, many women don't feel any desire to have sex with their husbands.

Lack of desire in women can be due to many different reasons. Often it is due to the physiology of aging as we go through menopause and lose our internal testosterone and sex drive, as well as our clitoral arousal cells required for an orgasm. Sometimes it is because we are in a relationship mismatch between our evolved mating strategies and the mate we have, resulting in subconscious (or conscious) desire for a "higher quality male." Issues in our relationship and environment can impact our libido, say, if we are under high levels of stress at work or if we have built up resentment in our relationship. And sometimes lack of desire is just an acceptance of defeat when we haven't been able to get the sex right with our partner and so have been unable to feel pleasure.

If you are suffering from HSDD, you need to ask yourself two very important private questions.

> 1) Is this a lifelong lack of interest in sex, or is it a lack of desire linked to a life change, such as medication, menopause or anger at your partner?

> 2) Do you *never* feel turned on or just not when you are

having sex with your partner? If reading *Fifty Shades* made you wet, or you enjoy fantasizing about your neighbor, it may not be your sex drive that is the issue. In this case, this is a critical factor to admit to yourself so that you can make the best decisions about your life.

Writing down very specifically when and where you have felt desire throughout your life and over the past week can help you and any clinician that you work with. This is the first step in discovering the cause for your lack of desire and whether sexual desire is something you want to find (or find again) in your life. If you feel the onset of a lack of sexual desire during the menopause transition, please know that you are not alone. This change is biologic and 100% normal. However, you can also decide if you want to feel this way. Testosterone supplementation through a prescription product can help inspire your sex drive—although you may be surprised to find out that (as of this writing) these medications are all currently prescribed "off-label," meaning they are not approved in the U.S. for use in women to counter poor libido. Given that testosterone supplementation is approved in many other Western countries, one can't help but wonder why none has yet been made available in America.

Fights Over the Female Viagra

The search for a Viagra-like drug to help women become aroused more quickly and easily seemed to start off with high hopes in 1998 when the male counterpart was launched on the market. After my struggles with sex when I was younger, I knew that this medication was going to be a huge blessing for many women who felt frustrated by their slow ability to become aroused or to orgasm. I, and many other sex scientists, watched in surprise as a cultural battle over women's sexuality developed around this issue—one that has managed, so far, to stop approval of any drugs that would help women who want better sexual function.

In a nutshell, the arguments against a female Viagra (cited by many feminists and natural product proponents, many of whom I respect in other areas of women's health) have been that: 1) the female sexual response is too complex to be treated medically; 2) since half of women feel low desire and don't regularly orgasm during vaginal intercourse, the condition is "normal" and not pathological; and 3) pharmaceutical companies are trying to "sell" a disease (for example, as seen in the 2013 news headline *"Female Sexual Dysfunction: A Case of Pharma Disease Mongering"*).

Let's look at these briefly. In fact, women who feel sexual desire when they read books or work with their personal trainer but not during sex with their spouse probably don't have a disease. They are more likely just experiencing ancient mating strategies and may benefit sexually from a new partner. Likewise, women whose lovers don't know how to touch them in a way to arouse them (so they can get turned on and feel desire during partnered sex) also aren't ill. In these ways, yes, female sexual function and orgasm is complex, and a pill may not be the "best" answer for these ladies.

But in another way these anti-female-Viagra folks are wrong. Even though well over half of us are near or far sighted, it doesn't make the condition "normal," and in fact it results in over 60% of us wearing corrective lenses to improve the condition (the fact that a lot of people suffer from something doesn't prevent us from trying to help with the problem). Some women who just aren't turned on by their partners would like to be (even just a little) so they could stay in the marriages they have. And many women want to respond more quickly and have more intense orgasms from the sex they are having. Most of us with jobs, kids and/or aging parents don't always want 20-plus-minute episodes of penile-vaginal intercourse or prolonged foreplay sessions (as some sex experts call for) in order to orgasm every time we have sex.

Female sexual dysfunction is not a "made up condition." We *know* that aging changes, stress, medications and disease all negatively impact a woman's sexual response, just like they impact a man's erection and sexual function. And we know that sex steroids or other medications can be used to combat these changes. There are 26 FDA-approved drugs for men to help them stay active and satisfied in bed. Let's start approving the female versions for those of us who want them!

Of course, as you wait for a female version of Viagra, if you are in mid-life, hormone replacement protocols can be helpful to you. HRT with testosterone has been proven in Level 1 studies (the highest quality evidence) to keep women's enjoyment of sex high. More than six million women in the U.S. currently use testosterone through off label prescriptions...while we wait for the FDA to catch up with the reality that we are living and having sex longer than ever.

Radical Center Ruminations - A recent editorial by Dr. Irwin Goldstein (Editor-in-Chief of the Journal of Sexual Medicine) said it best: "I want to vomit every time I hear someone say men's sexual health is so simple and women's so complicated." His statement was in response to the FDA's seeming inability to approve any sexual enhancement medications for women. In spite of the $1.5 billion being spent to develop safe and effective medications for women who want better sexual experiences, not one drug has yet been approved. (I hope as you are reading this book this sad statistic has changed.) Dr. Goldstein finishes his article by stating, "A government of the people, by the people and for the people has to eliminate gender bias in sexual health."

We need to demand that the "politics" in drug approval for women's sexuality be stopped. If medications demonstrate improvements for women, and side effect rates are equivalent to that of male counterparts, the drugs should be approved for women who want to take them. Peoples' marriages and happiness literally depend on it.

While hubby and I were busily working on keeping our love life alive during perimenopause, my reproductive tract started into its final death spiral, suddenly requiring my full attention. I needed to get serious in deciding how I would handle menopause and optimize my future sexual function and health in the second half of my life.

Chapter 15

The Right Stuff

Finally, in 2010, I drew the big hormonal "Pass Go" card into menopause as I had an emergency total hysterectomy *and* started hormone replacement all in the course of one week. Following constant bleeding and cramping during the holidays and a large family reunion in Hawaii with all our kids and their significant others, I needed medical attention STAT. Dr. Smetana rushed me in for surgery right after the New Year. But first, she and I sat down to draft my hormone replacement therapy (HRT) plan. Luckily, I had finally been doing some research on my own before my need for hormones became a medical emergency. At the time I had my ovaries (and therefore most of my sex steroids) removed in 2010, most women were completely confused about what to do for hormone replacement during menopause. A common response to the indecipherable chaos in the medical literature was just to ignore it all and go through the change as most women have throughout history, without medical intervention.

The problem with this approach is that we ladies are now living *four* times longer than our prehistoric ancestresses. Life expectancy for women between 200,000 and 20,000 B.C. was 20 years of age. These women would pop out a few children and then pass on. In the year 1 A.D. average female life expectancy was still only 28 years. By 1800 it had risen to 35. In 1900 things really started improving with an average life expectancy of 50 and women finally living to the point that menopause (average age of 51) was even an issue. Now since 2000, most women live to age 80 or beyond. We suddenly have half of our lives to live from the onset of premenopausal symptoms in our 40s to when we die. All of this being lived naturally with decreased levels of sex steroids and the health complications this causes. The only way to keep our brain and body cells bathed in the sex steroids with which they were created to function is to replace these hormones from an outside source. But how we replace these sex steroids is very important. Not all methods of hormone replacement are equal.

Making Sense of Menopause Hormones

I had my cervix, uterus and ovaries removed in January of 2010. This date was nearing the end of a very dark and confusing decade for Women's Health. We will look at how we got to where we are, most importantly so we can avoid going there again in the future. But first, I want to make sure that everyone—including those that are not yet menopausal and are thinking they can skip this chapter—understands a few basics about HRT.

- All sex steroid replacement hormones are not the same.

When you hear about "bad" pharmaceutical hormones, most of the data you are hearing referenced is from large studies (i.e., the Women's Health Initiative and the Heart and Estrogen/Progestin Replacement Study). Both of these studies used older style HRT, including oral estrogens collected from horse urine (conjugated equine estrogen) and an older progesterone product (MAP) that had been around since 1956. Newer and safer transdermal (skin) patches and modern generation progesterone products differ profoundly in their metabolism and safety from these older products. In fact, a recent article in the journal *Circulation* stated that safety data from these studies *"are not necessarily relevant"* to other types of hormone protocols.

• Data from older style HRT are widely extrapolated and used in American healthcare decision-making.

The current position paper by a leading North American menopausal organization gives the Women's Health Initiative (WHI) data with these older HRT protocols "prominent consideration." And a recent 2013 Cochrane Database Review (the final word on medical evidence) stated that *seventy percent* of this paper's results on the safety of long-term hormone replacement were derived from these studies. Additionally, both the NIH and the FDA discuss hormone replacement safety (in general) using data from these older hormone regimens. Plus they mix and match safety of hormones delivered by different routes in a manner that is not supported by data. Specifically, the FDA states that "The risks and benefits may be the same for all hormone products for menopause, such as pills, patches, vaginal creams, gels, rings..." In reality, the data is overwhelmingly suggestive of superior safety of newer generation estrogen and progesterone products applied to the skin.

• Taken together, women in America are undersold the benefit of hormone replacement for their overall health and are oversold the risks of HRT with the use of modern preparations.

"Bioidentical hormones" refers to both new FDA-approved hormone products and prescriptions compounded by a pharmacist. The term *bioidentical hormones* refers to hormone products that are chemically similar to the hormones our bodies make (e.g., human estrogen and not that from horse urine). Suzanne Somers, in her bestselling books over the past decade, introduced women to bioidentical hormone replacement that was individualized to each woman and that functioned more naturally with the sex steroid receptors in our bodies. Her desire to help women take charge of their menopause created a backlash from many in the medical community against the term "bioidentical." But recent data shows that Suzanne was correct (as she was about eating fewer carbs and more fat!). Many bioidentical hormone products are now FDA approved (including the products I use). You can see a current list of these in her recent book *I'm Too Young for This!* Individually compounded bioidenticals (speaking of course about those containing exact concentrations and purities of hormones) have been shown to improve health and quality of life for women in various stages of menopause. In fact, in one study, bioidentical hormones worked twice as well as conventional hormones for improving sexual dysfunction associated with menopause—likely because most compounded bioidentical protocols have testosterone in them, whereas many women on conventional HRT don't receive this critical hormone for best sexual function.

It is important to note that there is no Level 1 evidence that bioidentical hormones compounded by a pharmacist are safer or more effective than newer generation HRT pharmaceuticals (which are essentially also bioidentical). But the concept of measuring and tracking an individual's existing hormones levels through serial blood tests and replacing what needs replaced over time makes sense to me empirically. I am intrigued to see that the Forever Health™ website (*foreverhealth.com*) helps link people around the country with laboratories that can do general health blood testing (including hormone assays), which can then be shared with your physician. This website can also link patients with physicians who adhere to this more individualized approach to HRT.

After a decade of hormone chaos, people are opting for much more self-taught and self-directed methods to receive the health care they deserve. Sadly, time and time again I have seen symptoms of hormone disruption in women (and men) and suggested that these people go in to talk to a doctor about HRT. What I most commonly heard back, however, was that their doctor acted like they wanted a prescription for crack-cocaine rather than for approved, efficacious HRT. This isn't right, and it isn't evidence driven. It is also in direct contradiction to the ways that doctors treat themselves and their families.

One of the biggest indicators of the efficacy and safety of hormones for women going through menopause is to look at how female doctors or doctors' spouses deal with HRT. Over 70% of woman gynecologists or female partners of male gynecologists use hormones to navigate menopause. This compares to only 11% of the general U.S. population of women who choose hormones. That is truly an amazing difference! To understand this divide between patients and doctors, let's look at the history and politics of HRT.

The Politics of HRT

In July 2002, the Women's Health Initiative (WHI) made a dramatic public announcement suggesting a link between HRT and increases in heart attack, stroke and breast cancer in menopausal women. I still remember seeing the headlines at my work desk. Like perhaps everyone else, I worried for women; however, once I looked at the actual study, I was concerned in a different way. Specifically, the headlines burning through the media seemed to overstate the negative study data and completely ignored study findings of the benefits for women on HRT.

We will look at the actual data in a moment, but what you need to know about this study now, a decade later, is that it caused millions of women to stop or never start HRT. And sadly, this hormone hysteria got it wrong. The study investigators themselves have since withdrawn many of their findings, saying this study has caused needless suffering. The design and analysis have become so suspect that the founder of the North American Menopause Society has asked for an independent inquiry into the billion-dollar study. The saddest thing in all this bad medicine is the actual harm it has caused women. Estimates are that the millions of women who stopped or never began HRT after this study have had more than 43,000 annual bone fractures and even more yearly cardiovascular events (the leading cause of death in women). An entire generation of women, those with one of the longest projected life expectancies in human history, stopped HRT because of *one* study.

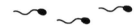

The headlines many people saw in 2002 regarding the WHI said something like **"Hormone replacement therapy associated with a 38% increase in stroke risk."** But let's look more closely at this study so we can arm ourselves against similar situations in the future (such as the current discussion regarding testosterone supplementation for men).

The 38% increase in the headline represented the *relative risk* of an increase in stroke for women taking HRT. Relative risk differences are when we compare the ratio of one probability to another—such as comparing a 1% rate to a 2% rate. Here the relative risk increase would be 100%. The more appropriate way to look at medical outcomes is to look at the *absolute risk (or actual risk)* difference from a treatment. For example, when comparing a 1% rate to a 2% rate, the absolute difference is 1%. In actuality, the absolute risk for stroke in the WHI study increased from **0.24%** (or 2.4 women per 10,000 treated) for women without HRT (placebo) to **0.33%** (or 3.3 women per 10,000 treated) in the HRT group. This represents a 0.09% absolute increase. That's right: *an increase of less than one-tenth of one percent caused these headlines!*

Another way of stating this data, which is actually more medically proper, is to frame the chance of *not* having the abnormal event or illness (in this case a stroke). Over 99% of women in this study did not have a stroke, regardless of their treatment. For women who did not take HRT, *99.76%* of them never had a stroke. In contrast, for women who used HRT, *99.67%* never had a stroke. Anyone can see that although the difference may have been statistically significant, if the data had been properly framed as an increase of 1 woman with a stroke out of 10,000 women, all of us over the past decade could have more accurately looked at overall benefits and risks of HRT.

Again, a valuable insight into the impact of this study can be seen in how physicians handled the information from this study. In contrast to the general population, among whom there was an 80% drop in the use of HRT, *only 8% of women in physician households stopped their hormone replacement for menopause.* This is because doctors knew that the overall quality of life and health benefits of HRT offset the risks for most women.

Do as I Do

When it came time for me to decide what to do about HRT as I got ready to say goodbye to my ovaries, I was lucky enough to have the following data points. I had read Suzanne Somers' books and knew I wanted bioidentical hormones as much as possible. (I see the eye rolling out there by some physicians, but she really does provide the most clear, concise information available on this topic.) I had also called several other female physician friends close to my age to compare notes. Almost without exception, they were following a protocol that included 1) removal of their entire reproductive tract (uterus and ovaries), 2) HRT with a bioidentical estrogen patch, 3) low dose testosterone (in a bimonthly injection) and 4) small vaginal tablets for local support of intimate tissues. All these women looked great and were physically active so I felt confident in that path.

Additionally, I knew that I could always stop taking hormones if I didn't like them, but that I couldn't always start HRT if I changed my mind years after menopause. Other than one small switch from a large generic estrogen patch to the small, clear Vivelle® patch, I have kept this same protocol ever since. And…I LOVE it!

The biggest surprise to me was how rapidly after starting the HRT I felt "normal" again in a way I hadn't felt in *years*. This first struck me several days after I was home from the hospital after my hysterectomy, lying on the couch yet again as I convalesced from another major surgery (my fifth in two years). This time I was full of energy and could multitask on the computer in a way I hadn't been capable of in a very long time. The best part was that once I was able to move around, I could go grocery shopping again without panic attacks. This anxiety is now a distant memory, although I can tell when I am due for my testosterone injection as I get a little nervous in the produce aisle (just kidding—sort of). I have since heard from other women that their menopause-related depression and anxiety also rapidly responded to HRT within days to weeks.

I look back now with gratitude that I had a very sharp Ob-Gyn who got me on the correct hormones right away. Menopause hits many women hard, the way it hit me. But remember that all this "craziness" is due to a biochemical shortage of sex steroids, like estrogen and testosterone, which we make in the first half of our lives. Once our reproductive capacity is over, these sex steroid losses wreak havoc in our bodies and brains even though we still have *HALF* of our lives to live. We are literally living a new phase in human sexual evolution, one woman at a time.

Hooray for Hormones

As you decide on whether HRT is right for you or someone you know, let's review the current international medical recommendations published in 2013. The most lay-friendly recommendations are those of the British Menopause Society. Sadly, the American consensus guidelines are still somewhat mired in politics around the WHI and are also not up to date.

These global guidelines suggest that for women under 60 or within 10 years from menopause, HRT benefits outweigh risks for:

- treating body changes such as itching, hot flashes and night sweats;

- some forms of depression;

- sexual dysfunction, including desire and orgasm (especially with testosterone added in);

- urination frequency and urgency problems;

- preventing osteoporosis-related fractures in at-risk women; and

- *decreasing coronary heart disease and all causes of mortality.*

A few general things to know about HRT include the following:

- Estrogen alone can be used in women after hysterectomy, but progesterone needs to be added if you still have a uterus.

- The risk of stroke and venous thromboembolism increases with *oral* HRT, but absolute risk is low before 60. In all cases, risk of stroke is lower with the estrogen patch.

- The risk of breast cancer in women over 50 on HRT is complex, but absolute risk is small. Increased risk may be associated with progesterone addition (which is needed if you still have a uterus).

- **If you have had surgical menopause and your ovaries have been removed, HRT should be used until *at least* the age of average menopause (i.e., 51)**

- HRT use in breast cancer survivors is not recommended at this time.

Overall, HRT makes sense for most women who start on the therapy before age 60. For these women, data suggest that it may actually lead to fewer heart attacks, less death and even less breast cancer. Watch for an avalanche of data over the next few years as women rack up years on the bioidentical hormones and continued safety reports come in. Also, many women will end up insisting like me that no one can take away their HRT. I thank my testosterone fairies every time I have a fabulous orgasm during hot sex with my hubby at 55 years of age!

Here are the overall concepts your doctor should follow when talking to you about HRT (adapted from the British Menopause Society recommendations):

- The choice to use HRT should be made by **each woman.**

- HRT dosage, regimen and duration should be **individualized,** with an annual review of **pros and cons.**

- **Arbitrary limits** should not be placed on duration of HRT.

- HRT started before 60 has a favorable benefit/risk profile and can prevent long-term health conditions with personal, social and economic burdens.

Contrast these global recommendations for HRT with U.S. federal agencies, such as the FDA and the NIH, recommending (as of this writing) that "Hormones should be used at the lowest dose that helps and for the shortest time." What does that mean, and how does that incorporate the findings of decreased disease and better quality of life for women using HRT? Global groups have called for the FDA to update this antiquated view which makes HRT sound like a toxin. If you have no medical contraindications but your doctor pushes you not to take HRT or if you are told to stop HRT after only a few years (and you aren't having health problems with it), please, please get a second opinion. Sometimes it is hard to find the right doctor, but HRT is a huge decision that will impact the *entire* second half of your life! It is worth researching and getting several opinions while <u>you</u> decide what is right for you.

More Ways to Ensure a Great Orgasm

While I rely on the testosterone part of my HRT to help me with sex drive and sexual function at my age, I also practice some other tricks of sexual science. If you are midlife or older (especially if you are menopausal) you may need these tricks.

Forget your body image for an hour

I sometimes have low self-esteem regarding my body. I can get distracted if I see my belly pouch while on top during intercourse. Or I worry if my heels are cracked and rough (and unsexy) during sex. In fact, 30% of women in heterosexual relationships say that their body image negatively impacts their sexual function. One interesting study found that if women masturbated in a room by themselves in front of a mirror, even if they had a negative body image, they got turned on and orgasmed more readily than they did with a partner. This study suggested that the sexual squelching aspect of the negative image wasn't due to their bodies and seeing them during sex but rather was due to concerns about how they appeared to their partner.

Let's remember, men want sex! It's likely that he isn't nearly as hung up about your body as you are...if you just keep having sex with him. And, as we've discussed, that can lead to more fun for you too.

Use your romance novels, favorite movies,
even porn to get turned on

If the chapter you are reading in your book is making you horny, *do not* turn the page. Unplug the distractions and go for it. Many younger women don't prefer and frankly don't need pornography or erotica, but it is very normal to become more interested in trying these stimulators as you age. Keep your sense of humor and be honest if scenes make you hot or not. If they are just grossing you out or making you laugh, turn it off!

Work on his erection

Seventy-five percent of women say that their sexual fulfillment increased when their man had a strong erection from pharmaceutical assistance. There is a reason erectile dysfunction drugs are so popular! For the aging male, erectile dysfunction medications don't just ensure he has an erection, but they can also help increase the overall size of the erection. Surveys show that women are often the drivers, asking their husbands to use ED meds for the very fact that women like the better erection! Remember, women are hard-wired to enjoy bigger and better.

Men's penile body changes happen slowly, and you may not be noticing a loss in the size and hardness of his erection until one day you realize, "Wow, he is different than before." Have him try some ED meds if appropriate. It is absolutely normal for him as he ages to have issues with erections. Part of your job will be to protect your orgasm by protecting his. In fact, let's look a bit more at how we can keep this part of our men going strong.

Erectile Dysfunction Science

Approximately 30 million U.S. men have erectile dysfunction (ED). ED increases with age so that half of men over 60 have some erectile issues. It is a mistake for us to assume that ED is just about sex. It is also an early warning sign for heart disease and diabetes. In particular, for the one in four ED patients who are under age 40, underlying diseases need to be ruled out early on. Even sexually inactive men who are not concerned if they have an erection for sex should go in for a diabetes check if they experience a lack of morning erections and sexual desires.

ED is most commonly treated with PDE-5 inhibitors such as Viagra®. These meds require only a limited physical exam to receive a prescription. But...poor response to these medications occurs in 30-50% of men, usually because of the man having low testosterone. PDE-5 inhibitors only reach their full potential when a man's internal testosterone levels are normal. In fact, testosterone levels are so highly related to ED that European guidelines include testosterone testing for ALL men presenting with ED. ED happens as the man ages and his testosterone levels drop. These changes result in a loss of smooth muscle cells in the penis and an increase in connective tissue and fat cell deposits.

Over time it is common for PDE-5 inhibitors alone to stop working. If you or your partner is experiencing this, see if it helps to add testosterone therapy along with the Viagra. If you are a young man with ED and trying to conceive, do *not* take testosterone. It can act as a contraceptive!

Erectile function is highly correlated with exercise. Specifically, the risk of severe ED decreases 83% with exercise that burns 3,000 kcals per week. All exercise helps—walking, jogging and tennis all put men at lower risk. Just 3-4 hours per week of exercise can decrease ED by half. And of course one of the best things you can do for ED is to have more frequent ejaculation. In a study with 60-year-old men, those having sex three times a week or more had only a quarter of the cases of ED as the men in the group having intercourse less than once a week. Use it or lose it!

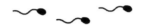

Aging brings changes for both men and women in our physical health and our sexual function. As much as we joke about people trying to stay young at any cost, the truth is that medications can allow people to keep enjoying sexual intimacy for decades beyond our natural arc of life. It is interesting to remember that even though we are living much longer than humans previously lived, our reproductive life span has not changed. So there is no evolutionary pressure on our species to prolong sex steroid secretion and delay menopause or the male equivalent "andropause." The only solution, for now, is to replace these hormones so that our cells that allow intimacy, pleasure and orgasm remain alive and well. Before we leave this section on hormones, let's briefly touch base on andropause, or late-onset hypogonadism, in men.

Andropause – The Other Half of the Pair

While women are going through the rocky road of menopause, their male partners are often going through their own hormonal shift called *andropause*. Andropause starts in a man's 40s as his testosterone levels begin to decline by 2% a year. This may not seem like a lot, but it can add up over 20, 30 or even 40 years. This sex steroid, testosterone, provides both men and women with their sexual desire. As men age, decreasing testosterone (T) levels can leave men feeling apathetic about sex. It is important to clarify that although erectile dysfunction drugs, such as Viagra®, can help a man have a harder, more certain erection, these types of medication do not improve sexual desire. If a man rarely wants sex because of changes in T due to aging, all the Viagra in the world may not help this. And decreasing T in aging men is not just about sex, it can also result in degenerative body and mind changes, similar to those we see in menopausal woman (through similar mechanisms).

The medical names for low T include *late-onset hypogonadism* or *androgen deficiency in the aging male*. Men with this condition tend to have a classic history: a declining mojo, the proverbial beer belly, using Viagra at home (but it isn't working as well anymore), development of diabetes and starting on Lipitor® for high cholesterol. And many of these men will receive bad advice from physicians who really don't understand andropause. Diagnosis of and treatment planning for low T should be done with physicians who are up to date on this rapidly changing field and whose credentials and medical society memberships include the terms "aging male" or "sexual medicine." These specialists can better interpret T blood levels as well as ensure men take the "Aging Male" ADAM survey to screen symptoms for correct diagnosis. Forever Health™ can also help men get a blood test and find a physician who specializes in aging male problems.

Symptoms of Andropause

The current physician guidelines suggest that low T be considered in *all midlife or older men* who are symptomatic for any of the following:

- Low libido

- Poor or infrequent morning erections (less than three a week)

- Erectile dysfunction

- Depressed mood and/or fatigue

- Cognitive impairment (poor performance at work)

- Insulin resistance

- Obesity

- Metabolic syndrome

- Diabetes mellitus type 2

- Decreased muscle mass and strength

- Decreased bone mineral density and osteoporosis

- Decreased vitality

- Vitamin D deficiency

- On glucocorticoids (such as prednisone or Kenalog®)

- On narcotics (such as hydrocodone)

Men who have any of these symptoms or conditions should have a testosterone blood test done. You can learn more at my Sex, Science and Nature site or at the International Society for the Study of the Aging Male (ISSAM) on the correct time and type of blood test for low T, as well as on what are normal levels of T.

Another symptom of andropause that is just beginning to be understood is that of *irritable male syndrome*. These are men who react to the declining T of andropause with a complete personality change. They become very critical and mean. Men with this syndrome may actually become worse for a bit on T therapy, but in the long run reactivity and irrational anger can be better controlled on T. Dr. Jed Diamond's book *Mr. Mean: Saving Your Relationship from the Irritable Male Syndrome* can be a great resource to understand this condition.

Having low T can decrease a man's quality of life, his sex life and even his lifespan. A lot is at stake here. Low T can increase the risk of cardiovascular disease and severe, treatment-resistant depression. In fact, there is a strong link between low T and suicide rates in older men. Remember that persistent use of corticosteroids (such as prednisone or Kenalog® for asthma or arthritis) can dramatically lower T levels, as can narcotics (opiates) and marijuana. Recent evidence also suggests that statins (such as Lipitor®) may decrease T levels. Men who are on these medications should be proactive about having their T levels tested.

In spite of the very real beneficial impact on men's health and lives that T therapy can provide, millions of men remain undiagnosed and untreated for this condition. This is because a blood test alone cannot necessarily diagnose low T. The blood test must be combined with the Aging Male survey. If your doctor doesn't provide you with the ADAM survey or do the correct blood test for T, find a different doctor. *Men who are obese and do not have low testosterone but who have positive symptoms on the survey may benefit from a three-month trial on T therapy.* The ISSAM suggests that men with a hematocrit (proportion, by volume, of the blood that consists of red blood cells) of over 52%, untreated obstructive sleep apnea, or untreated congestive heart failure may not be treated with T without resolution of these issues first.

Radical Center Ruminations- Getting accurate information and advice regarding the safety of T therapy for men just got a lot harder. Two recent observational studies have made quite a splash in the news. Researchers in both these studies looked back at peoples' medical records to observe their health outcomes in order to see if they had been taking T and if so, whether the medication increased their chances of stroke, heart attack or death. These studies suggested they did. However, observational studies like these provide low-level evidence for medical outcomes. Additionally, these studies did not control adequately for the fact that men taking testosterone have sex and exercise more than those that don't. Both sex and exercise increase a man's chance of heart attack substantially, but they both make life much more worth living! Each man needs to weigh these risks and benefits for himself.

Unfortunately, the FDA has really latched on to these studies, driven in large part by pressure from the group Public Citizen founded by Ralph Nader. Specifically, an FDA advisory review panel recommended that testosterone therapy not be used in aging men with low T. I am frankly amazed at the FDA's reaction to these specific studies and their failure to look at the much broader science and medical expert guidelines on the overall benefits of testosterone therapy in aging men, including improved quality of life.

Numerous medical societies have come out strongly opposed to the media and regulatory hysteria over these studies, discussing the weakness of the cited data. The term hormonaphobia has even been coined to describe the frenzy around these two studies reminiscent of the menopause HRT debate a decade ago. Specifically these new testosterone studies included heavily manipulated statistics (one study used a proprietary software program and was published by the statistical software company's employees). Oddly, FDA and the media have overemphasized these studies and ignored the regular and ongoing publication of higher quality studies showing an overall benefit of T therapy, including improved health and enjoyment of life.

If you (as either an aging man or a woman) have benefited from hormone replacement, let the FDA know your story and also ask your doctor to show support for letting people **choose** from these largely beneficial medications used by millions of people around the world to feel and function better during the second half of their lives.

Both andropause and menopause require our attention and self education, as well as an expectation of informed dialogue with our healthcare providers. These people shouldn't tell us *what* we should do, they should tell us what the benefits and risks are of different options so that we feel comfortable deciding what our best choice is for this exciting time in life.

Chapter 16

Upward And Onward

Life was much better all the way around at our house and at Bio after I started my hormone replacement. With two new contract manufacturers helping us meet our growing inventory needs, Pre-Seed was ready to move into the national drugstore chains, and we did so smoothly and quickly. More independent studies were published showing Pre-Seed's safety and efficacy. This led to Pre-Seed being mentioned as a lubricant of choice for fertility patients in medical guidelines and textbooks (see *preseed. com* for a review of these).

In a public health victory, based in part on our communications with the FDA, labeling of personal lubricants that were not sperm-safe changed to become more accurate. We had spent over ten years trying to raise awareness of the possible harm to sperm from lubricants and, finally, perseverance paid off. These everyday lubricants were no longer able to claim on their package that they were "nonspermicidal." Now these lubricants are required to clarify that they "Do not contain a spermicide," which means they are not contraceptive drugs.

And in my favorite science surprise of all, data from the prestigious Magee-Womens Research Institute reported that Pre-Seed's isotonic formula was safe for the fragile cells of intimacy, whereas common high osmolarity lubricants caused damage to these cells. Through this study, our goal of sexual advocacy was furthered beyond helping TTC couples; now, Pre-Seed's formula was being promoted for *any* couple wanting to have enjoyable nonirritating sexual pleasure and, most important to me, *sexual bonding.*

Our success with Pre-Seed led to several "suitors" knocking on our door, as companies approached us with interest in buying Pre-Seed. Finally, in October of 2012 Gil and I knew it was time to let our "baby," Pre-Seed, grow up and out of our protective arms. It was time for Pre-Seed to become part of an established product line in a larger women's healthcare company. And it was time for me to start focusing on my health much more fully than I had been able to.

After celebrations and transitional work to move Pre-Seed to its new home, I was able to have a long delayed back fusion surgery to better manage the constant pain in my right ankle and foot. I also changed my diet to a "Paleo" diet, at the urging of my arthritis specialist and my orthopedic surgeon, in response to the autoimmune arthritis I had developed during my years of chronic pain and health problems. In general, I sought to refocus my life on improving my health, decreasing my stress and enjoying our boys' growth and my husband's love. I'm happy to say that after the surgery *the pain I had been having in my right leg was gone,* and sensation returned to my right foot for the first time in five years!

During the month after my surgery, with no more pain and healthy eating, amazingly, my world began to fill with colors again. I hadn't even realized that the unremitting pain and stress I'd been feeling had made me "color blind"—my world had gone "gray." Once the colors returned and with a new lease on life, I began to write down the story of my journey through life and sex as a woman and the tale of my bumpy ride to "conceive" and market Pre-Seed. Yet, always the educator, I interlaced throughout these stories some of what I have learned—from personal and professional experience and from the laboratory and literature—about the amazing and often misunderstood world of sex, science and nature. I hope I've been able to open up more "colorful" worlds of sexuality for others through my research and products, my successes and failures, and my review of the science of sex.

As I look back, I believe all my adventures in love, marriage, science and business have in some way been about exploring the depths of sexuality so that I could understand it from the inside out. For me, few activities in this life have brought me as much joy as sex—the act of sex, the children I gained from sex, the business I built from sex, the lovers I loved through sex and the husband I adore through sex.

Whatever your journey has been through the mystery of sex, I hope for you to see new and wider paths on your future travels, roads no longer paved with fears about sex but instead with communication, technique, advocacy and new ideas about intimacy. Sexuality is that part of us linked most clearly to our distant human past. As such, it is powerful in us like few other aspects of ourselves. Let's take control of our sexuality and enliven the mystery of sex for ourselves again and again.

Thank you for joining me on my unique journey. I hope it helps you look at your own with a better understanding and even compassion, mixed in with a renewed sense of excitement for the future. You can visit *sexscienceandnature.com* for updates on the science of sex and tips on understanding the newest medical research. I also look forward to hearing your comments, stories and questions about sex and intimacy.

Turn off the TV. Try something new. Get the medical help you need to create the sexual script and fulfillment you long for. Remember what turned you on about your partner. Surprise them and yourself with a new sense of joy and fearlessness in the bedroom or on a trail in the woods.

Let me know how it is going, and I will do the same with you all as we each move forward on life's path with the people we love.

Blessings-

Dr. E

Bibliography

Acevedo BP, Aron A, Fisher HE, Brown LL. Neural correlates of long-term intense romantic love. *Soc Cogn Affect Neurosci.* 2012;7:145-59.

Adriaens E, Remon JP. Mucosal irritation potential of personal lubricants relates to product osmolality as detected by the slug mucosal irritation assay. *Sex Transm Dis.* 2008;35:512-6.

Agarwal A, Deepinder F, Cocuzza M, Short RA, Evenson DP. Effect of vaginal lubricants on sperm motility and chromatin integrity: a prospective comparative study. *Fertil Steril.* 2008;89:375–9.

Althof SE, McMahon CG, Waldinger MD, et al. An update of the International Society of Sexual Medicine's guidelines for the diagnosis and treatment of premature ejaculation (PE). *J Sex Med.* 201411:1392-422.

American College of Obstetricians and Gynecologists Committee on Gynecologic Practice; American Society for Reproductive Medicine Practice Committee. Compounded bioidentical menopausal hormone therapy. *Fertil Steril.* 2012;98:308-12.

Anderson GL, Limacher M, Assaf AR, et al. Women's Health Initiative Steering Committee. Effects of conjugated equine estrogen in postmenopausal women with hysterectomy: the Women's Health Initiative randomized controlled trial. *JAMA.* 2004;291:1701-12.

Association of Reproductive Health Professionals. Female Sexual Response. [Clinical Fact Sheet]. http://www.arhp.org/publications-and-resources/clinical-fact-sheets/female-sexual-response . 2008. Accessed September 5, 2014.

Barash D, Lipton J. *The Myth of Monogamy: Fidelity and Infidelity in Animals and People.* New York: Henry Holt and Company; 2001.

Basaria S, Coviello AD, Travison TG, et al. Adverse events associated with testosterone administration. *N Engl J Med.* 2010;363:109-22.

Basson R, Leiblum S, Brotto L, et al. Revised definitions of women's sexual dysfunction. *J Sex Med*. 2004;1:40-8.

Basson R. The recurrent pain and sexual sequelae of provoked vestibulodynia: a perpetuating cycle. *J Sex Med*. 2012;9:2077-92.

Begay O, Jean-Pierre N, Abraham CJ, et al. Identification of personal lubricants that can cause rectal epithelial cell damage and enhance HIV type 1 replication in vitro. *AIDS Res Hum Retroviruses*. 2011;27:1019-24.

Bell AV, Hinde K, Newson L. Who was helping? The scope for female cooperative breeding in early Homo. *PLoS One*. 2013 Dec 18;8(12):e83667.

Berger ML, Martin BC, Husereau D, et al. A questionnaire to assess the relevance and credibility of observational studies to inform health care decision making: an ISPOR-AMCP-NPC Good Practice Task Force report. *Value Health*. 2014;17:143-56.

Bethea CL, Reddy AP, Tokuyama Y, Henderson JA, Lima FB. Protective actions of ovarian hormones in the serotonin system of macaques. *Front Neuroendocrinol*. 2009;30:212-38.

Bettinger JA, Celentano DD, Curriero FC, Adler NE, Millstein SG, Ellen JM. Does parental involvement predict new sexually transmitted diseases in female adolescents? *Arch Pediatr Adolesc Med*. 2004;158:666-70.

Biglia N, Ujcic E, Kubatzki F, et al. Personal use of hormone therapy by postmenopausal women doctors and male doctors' wives in Italy after the publication of WHI trial. *Maturitas*. 2006;54:181-92.

Bobrow M. *Views from the Tightrope: Living Wisely in an Uncertain World*. Burdett, NY: Larson Publishing; 1997.

Boonstra HD, Nash E. A Surge of State Abortion Restrictions Puts Providers—and the Women They Serve—in the Crosshairs. *Guttmacher Policy Review*. 2014;17:9-15.

Bove R, Chitnis T, Houtchens M. Menopause in multiple sclerosis: therapeutic considerations. *J Neurol*. 2014;261:1257-68.

Brauer M, Lakeman M, van Lunsen R, Laan E. Predictors of Task-Persistent and Fear-Avoiding Behaviors in Women with Sexual Pain Disorders. *J Sex Med.* 2014 Sep 18. doi: 10.1111/jsm.12697.

Burger HG, MacLennan AH, Huang KE, Castelo-Branco C. Evidence-based assessment of the impact of the WHI on women's health. *Climacteric.* 2012;15:281-7.

Buvat J. Who would benefit from testosterone therapy? International Society for Sexual Medicine [Reviews and Reports]. http://www.issm.info/news/review-reports/who-would-benefit-from-testosterone-therapy. 2009 Accessed September 5, 2014.

Canonico M, Oger E, Plu-Bureau G, et. al; Estrogen and Thromboembolism Risk (ESTHER) Study Group. Hormone therapy and venous thromboembolism among postmenopausal women: impact of the route of estrogen administration and progestogens: the ESTHER study. *Circulation.* 2007;115:840-5.

Capogrosso P, Colicchia M, Ventimiglia E, et al. One patient out of four with newly diagnosed erectile dysfunction is a young man—worrisome picture from the everyday clinical practice. *J Sex Med.* 2013;10:1833-41.

Cappola AR. Testosterone therapy and risk of cardiovascular disease in men. *JAMA.* 2013;310:1805-6.

Carroll JC, Rosario ER. The potential use of hormone-based therapeutics for the treatment of Alzheimer's disease. *Curr Alzheimer Res.* 2012;9:18-34.

Cashdan E. Hormones, sex, and status in women. *Horm Behav.* 1995;29:354-66.

Castaneda C. *The Teachings of Don Juan: A Yaqui Way of Knowledge.* New York: Washington Square Press; 1985.

Castellanos, M. "Stop Saying Vagina (unless You Mean It)." http://www.thesexmd.com. http://www.thesexmd.com/stop-saying-vagina-unless-mean. September 6, 2014. Accessed September 12, 2014.

Chapman, J. *How to Lose Your Wife to Another Woman: A Memoir of a Mixed-Orientation Marriage.* CreateSpace Independent Publishing Platform. 2014.

Chiang, O. "Trojan: U.S. Market Size For Vibrators $1 Billion, Twice The Condom Market Size." Forbes Magazine. http://www.forbes.com/sites/oliverchiang/2011/01/07/trojan-us-market-size-for-vibrators-1-billon-twice-the-condom-market-size. 2011. Accessed September 5, 2014.

Chlebowski RT, Cirillo DJ, Eaton CB, et al. Estrogen alone and joint symptoms in the Women's Health Initiative randomized trial. *Menopause.* 2013;20:600-8.

Chung M, Raman G, Trikalinos T, Lau J, Ip S. Interventions in primary care to promote breastfeeding: an evidence review for the U.S. Preventive Services Task Force. *Ann Intern Med.* 2008;149:565-82.

Clarke T. FDA panel backs limiting use of testosterone replacement drugs. http://www.reuters.com/article/2014/09/17/usa-health-testosterone-idUSL1N0RI2V820140917. September 17, 2014. Accessed September 24, 2014.

Cody JD, Jacobs ML, Richardson K, Moehrer B, Hextall A. Oestrogen therapy for urinary incontinence in post-menopausal women. *Cochrane Database Syst Rev.* 2012 Oct 17;10:CD001405.

Cohen DA, Farley TA, Taylor SN, Martin DH, Schuster MA. When and where do youths have sex? The potential role of adult supervision. *Pediatrics.* 2002; 110:e66.

Comfort A, Quilliam S. *The Joy of Sex.* New York: Three Rivers Press. 2009.

Conley TD, Ziegler A, Moors AC, Matsick JL, Valentine B. A critical examination of popular assumptions about the benefits and outcomes of monogamous relationships. *Pers Soc Psychol Rev.* 2013;17:124-41.

Cook, John. "Former Top Exec of ING Fertility Files Suit." Seattlepi.com. http://www.seattlepi.com/business/article/Former-top-exec-of-ING-Fertility-files-suit-1133857.php . January 5, 2004. Accessed September 5, 2014.

Corona G, Rastrelli G, Maggi M. Diagnosis and treatment of late-onset hypogonadism: systematic review and meta-analysis of TRT outcomes. *Best Pract Res Clin Endocrinol Metab.* 2013;27:557-79.

Corona G, Vignozzi L, Sforza A, Maggi M. Risks and benefits of late onset hypogonadism treatment: an expert opinion. *World J Mens Health.* 2013;31:103-25.

Costa RM, Brody S. Women's relationship quality is associated with specifically penile-vaginal intercourse orgasm and frequency. *J Sex Marital Ther.* 2007;33:319-27.

Costa RM, Miller GF, Brody S. Women who prefer longer penises are more likely to have vaginal orgasms (but not clitoral orgasms): implications for an evolutionary theory of vaginal orgasm. *J Sex Med.* 2012;9:3079-88.

Crepaz N, Marks G, Liau A, et al.; HIV/AIDS Prevention Research Synthesis (PRS) Team. Prevalence of unprotected anal intercourse among HIV-diagnosed MSM in the United States: a meta-analysis. *AIDS.* 2009;23:1617-29.

Critelli JW, Bivona JM. Women's erotic rape fantasies: an evaluation of theory and research. *J Sex Res.* 2008;45:57-70.

Dahabreh IJ, Paulus JK. Association of episodic physical and sexual activity with triggering of acute cardiac events: systematic review and meta-analysis. *JAMA.* 2011;305:1225-33.

David SS, Blakeway J. *Making Babies: A Proven 3-Month Program for Maximum Fertility.* New York, NY; Little, Brown and Company: 2009.

Davis SR, Braunstein GD. Efficacy and safety of testosterone in the management of hypoactive sexual desire disorder in postmenopausal women. *J Sex Med.* 2012;9:1134-48.

de Villiers TJ, Pines A, Panay N, et al. International Menopause Society. Updated 2013 International Menopause Society recommendations on menopausal hormone therapy and preventive strategies for midlife health. *Climacteric.* 2013;16:316-37.

DeLecce TL, Polheber JP, Matchock RL. Sociosexual orientation and 2D:4D ratios in women: Relationship to men's desirability ratings as a long-term pair bond. *Arch Sex Behav.* 2014;43:319-27.

Devi G, Sugiguchi F, Pedersen AT, Abrassart D, Glodowski M, Nachtigall L. Current attitudes on self-use and prescription of hormone therapy among New York City gynaecologists. *Menopause Int.* 2013;19:121-6.

Dezzutti CS, Brown ER, Moncla B,et al. Is wetter better? An evaluation of over-the-counter personal lubricants for safety and anti-HIV-1 activity. *PLoS One.* 2012;7(11):e48328.

Diamond J. *Mr. Mean: Saving Your Relationship from the Irritable Male Syndrome.* San Rafael, CA: Vox Novus. 2010.

Diamond J. *Stress Relief For Men.* Berkely, CA: North Atlantic Books. 2014

Donders GG, Folens S, Peperstraete B, Bellen G. Age of sexual debut and central introital dyspareunia. *Eur J Obstet Gynecol Reprod Biol.* 2011;158:90-2.

Dreweke J. U.S. Abortion Rate Continues to Decline While Debate over Means to the End Escalates. *Guttmacher Policy Review.* 2014;17:2-7.

Durex. "2005 Global Sex Survey Results." http://data360.org/pdf/20070416064139.Global%20Sex%20Survey.pdf . Accessed September 5, 2014.

Ellington JE, Broemeling LD, Broder SJ, Jones AE, Choker DA, Wright RW. Comparison of fresh and cryopreserved human sperm attachment to bovine oviduct (Uterine tube) epithelial cells in vitro. *Jour of Andrology.* 1999;20:492-99.

Ellington JE, Carney EW, Farrell PB, Simkins ME, Foote RH. Bovine 1-2-cell embryo development using a simple medium in three oviduct epithelial cell co-culture systems. *Biol. of Reprod.* 1990;43:100-07.

Ellington JE, Evenson D, Rice G, Brisbois S, Hiss G, Jones A, Broder, S, Wright RW, Coculture of human sperm and bovine oviduct epithelial cells decreases sperm chromatin structural changes seen over time in culture. *Fertil Steril.* 1998;69:643-49.

Ellington JE, Ignotz GG, Ball BA, Meyers-Wallen VN, Currie WB. De novo protein synthesis by bovine uterine tube (oviduct) epithelial cells changes during co-culture with bull spermatozoa. *Biol. of Reprod.* 1993;48:851-56.

Ellington JE, Varner DD, Mathison P, et al. Interactions of stallion spermatozoa and mare uterine tube (oviduct) epithelial cells in a co-culture system. *Molecular Andrology* 1992;5:101-12.

Ellsworth RM, Bailey DH. Human female orgasm as evolved signal: a test of two hypotheses. *Arch Sex Behav.* 2013;42:1545-54.

Evenson, D. Sperm Chromatin Structure Assay (SCSA®): 30 years of experience with the SCSA®. In: *Sperm DNA and Male Infertility and ART*, Agarwal A, Springer Z, eds. Springer Publishers 2011.

Fallis EE, Rehman US, Purdon C. Perceptions of partner sexual satisfaction in heterosexual committed relationships. *Arch Sex Behav.* 2014;43:541-50.

Family Circle Magazine. Family Circle Survey: Mom Confessions. http://www.familycircle.com/health/emotional/self-improvement/family-circle-survey-mom-confessions/?ordersrc=rdfc1108470#page=3. March 2014. Accessed September 24, 2014.

Feneley MR, Carruthers M. Is testosterone treatment good for the prostate? Study of safety during long-term treatment. *J Sex Med.* 2012;9:2138-49.

Finkle WD, Greenland S, Ridgeway GK, et al. Increased risk of non-fatal myocardial infarction following testosterone therapy prescription in men. *PLoS One.* 2014;9(1):e85805.

Foldès P, Cuzin B, Andro A. Reconstructive surgery after female genital mutilation: a prospective cohort study. *Lancet.* 2012;380:134-41.

Ford CA, Pence BW, Miller WC, et al. Predicting adolescents' longitudinal risk for sexually transmitted infection: results from the National Longitudinal Study of Adolescent Health. *Arch Pediatr Adolesc* Med. 2005;159:657-64.

Frey BN, Dias RS. Sex hormones and biomarkers of neuroprotection and neurodegeneration: implications for female reproductive events in bipolar disorder. *Bipolar Disord.* 2014;16:48-57.

Fugl-Meyer KS, Oberg K, Lundberg PO, Lewin B, Fugl-Meyer A. On orgasm, sexual techniques, and erotic perceptions in 18- to 74-year-old Swedish women. *J Sex Med.* 2006;3:56-68.

Gangestad SW, Simpson JA, Cousins AJ, Garver-Apgar CE, Christensen PN. Women'spreferences for male behavioral displays change across the menstrual cycle. *Psychol Sci.* 2004;15:203-7.

Gaskin I. *Spiritual Midwifery* (4th ed.). Summertown, Tenn.: Book Pub Co. 2002.

Giles KR, McCabe MP. Conceptualizing women's sexual function: linear vs. circular models of sexual response. *J Sex Med.* 2009;6:2761-71.

Glaser R, Dimitrakakis C. Testosterone therapy in women: myths and misconceptions. *Maturitas.* 2013;74:230-4.

Glass J, Levchak P. Red states, blue states, and divorce: understanding the impact of conservative Protestantism on regional variation in divorce rates. *AJS.* 2014;119:1002-46.

Goldstein A, Pukall, Goldstein I. *When Sex Hurts: A Woman's Guide to Banishing Sexual Pain.* Boston: Da Capo Lifelong Books. 2011.

Goldstein I. Raising the Glass Ceiling: Not All "Men" are Created Equal. *J Sex Med.* 2014;11:1885-7.

Gori A, Giannini M, Craparo G, Caretti V, Nannini I, Madathil R, Schuldberg D. Assessment of the relationship between the use of birth control pill and the characteristics of mate selection. *J Sex Med.* 2014;11:2181-7.

Graziottin A, Serafini A. Depression and the menopause: why antidepressants are not enough? *Menopause Int.* 2009;15:76-81.

Greene B. *The Fabric of the Cosmos: Space, Time, and the Texture of Reality.* New York, NY: A.A. Knopf. 2004.

Greene RA. *Perfect Hormone Balance for Fertility: The Ultimate Guide to Getting Pregnant.* New York, NY: Clarkson Potter. 2007.

Gurian M. *The Purpose of Boys: Helping Our Sons Find Meaning, Significance, and Direction in Their Lives.* San Francisco, Calif.: Jossey-Bass. 2009.

Gurian M. *The Wonder of Boys.* 10th Anniversary Ed. New York, NY.: Tarcher. 2006.

Haavio-Mannila E, Kontula O. Correlates of increased sexual satisfaction. *Arch Sex Behav.* 1997;26:399-419.

Haddad RM, Kennedy CC, Caples SM, et al. Testosterone and cardiovascular risk in men: a systematic review and meta-analysis of randomized placebo-controlled trials. *Mayo Clin Proc.* 2007;82:29-39.

Hall KS, Moreau C, Trussell J. Young women's perceived health and lifetime sexual experience: results from the national survey of family growth. *J Sex Med.* 2012;9:1382-91.

Hamann S, Herman RA, Nolan CL, Wallen K. Men and women differ in amygdala response to visual sexual stimuli. *Nat Neurosci.* 2004;7:411-6.

Hanauer J, Hanauer J. *Red Hot Touch: A Head-to-Toe Handbook for Mind-Blowing Orgasms.* New York: Broadway. 2008.

Hayes RD, Bennett CM, Fairley CK, Dennerstein L. What can prevalence studies tell us about female sexual difficulty and dysfunction? *J Sex Med.* 2006;3:589-95.

Hayes RD. Circular and linear modeling of female sexual desire and arousal. *J Sex Res.* 2011;48:130-41.

Heffron R, Donnell D, Rees H, et al; Partners in Prevention HSV/HIV Transmission Study Team. Use of hormonal contraceptives and risk of HIV-1 transmission: a prospective cohort study. *Lancet Infect Dis.* 2012;12:19-26.

Heiman JR, Talley DR, Bailen JL, et al. Sexual function and satisfaction in heterosexual couples when men are administered sildenafil citrate (Viagra) for erectile dysfunction: a multicentre, randomised, double-blind, placebo-controlled trial. *BJOG.* 2007;114:437-47.

Henderson VW, St John JA, Hodis HN, et al. Cognition, mood, and physiological concentrations of sex hormones in the early and late postmenopause. *Proc Natl Acad Sci USA.* 2013;110:20290-5.

Henrich J, Boyd R, Richerson PJ. The puzzle of monogamous marriage. *Philos Trans R Soc Lond B Biol Sci.* 2012;367:657-69.

Herbenick D, Reece M, Sanders S, Dodge B, Ghassemi A, Fortenberry JD. Prevalence and characteristics of vibrator use by women in the United States: results from a nationally representative study. *J Sex Med.* 2009;6:1857-66.

Herbenick D, Reece M, Schick V, Sanders SA, Dodge B, Fortenberry JD. Sexual behaviors, relationships, and perceived health status among adult women in the United States: results from a national probability sample. *J Sex Med.* 2010;7 (Suppl 5):277-90.

Herbenick D. *Because It Feels Good: A Woman's Guide to Sexual Pleasure and Satisfaction.* Emmaus, Pa.: Rodale. 2009.

Hernández Martínez A, Pascual Pedreño AI, Baño Garnés AB, Melero Jiménez MR, Molina Alarcón M. [Differences in cesarean sections between spontaneous and induced labour]. *Rev Esp Salud Publica.* 2014;88:383-93.

Hess JA, Coffelt TA. Verbal communication about sex in marriage: patterns of language use and its connection with relational outcomes. *J Sex Res.* 2012;49:603-12.

Hochschild A, Machung A. *The Second Shift.* New York: Penguin Books. 2003.

Hogarth H, Ingham R. Masturbation among young women and associations with sexual health: an exploratory study. *J Sex Res.* 2009;46:558-67.

Iftikhar S, Shuster LT, Johnson RE, Jenkins SM, Wahner-Roedler DL. Use of bioidentical compounded hormones for menopausal concerns: cross-sectional survey in an academic menopause center. *J Womens Health (Larchmt).* 2011;20:559-65.

Impett EA, Peplau LA. Sexual compliance: gender, motivational, and relationship perspectives. *J Sex Res.* 2003;40:87-100.

Impett EA, Strachman A, Finkel EJ, Gable SL. Maintaining sexual desire in intimate relationships: the importance of approach goals. *J Pers Soc Psychol.* 2008;94:808-23.

International Menopause Society. Billion Dollar NIH Study May Have Harmed Women's Health – Call For An Independent Commission Of Enquiry [Press Release].. http://www.imsociety.org/pdf_files/comments_and_press_statements/ims_press_statement_05_07_12.pdf . 2012. Accessed September 5, 2014.

International Menopause Society. Ten years after the WHI, the IMS calls for NIH to revise recommendations on hormone replacement therapy (HRT). [Press Release]. http://www.imsociety.org/pdf_files/comments_and_press_statements/ims_press_statement_09_07_12.pdf. 2012. Accessed September 5, 2014.

International Society for the Study of Women's Sexual Health. New National Poll: American Women Object to Societal Gender Inequity Regarding Sexual Satisfaction, Treatment of Sexual Dysfunction. [Press Release]. http://www.prnewswire.com/news-releases/new-national-poll-american-women-object-to-societal-gender-inequity-regarding-sexual-satisfaction-treatment-of-sexual-dysfunction-242216881.html . 2014. Accessed September 5, 2014.

Isaacs AJ, Drew SV, McPherson K. UK women doctors' use of hormone replacement therapy: 10-year follow up. *Climacteric.* 2005;8:154-61.

Isley MM, Edelman A, Kaneshiro B, Peters D, Nichols MD, Jensen JT. Sex education and contraceptive use at coital debut in the United States: results from Cycle 6 of the National Survey of Family Growth. *Contraception.* 2010;82:236-42.

Jannini EA, Rubio-Casillas A, Whipple B, Buisson O, Komisaruk BR, Brody S. Female orgasm(s): one, two, several. *J Sex Med.* 2012;9:956-65.

James EL. *Fifty shades of Grey.* London; Vintage: 2011.

Jeffcoat H. *Sex Without Pain: A Self-Treatment Guide to the Sex Life You Deserve.* Los Angeles, CA.: Active Orange Publishing. 2014

Keramat A, Masoomi SZ, Mousavi SA, Poorolajal J, Shobeiri F, Hazavhei SM. Quality of life and its related factors in infertile couples. *J Res Health Sci.* 2014;14:57-63.

Kerner I, Raykeil H. *Love in the Time of Colic: The New Parents' Guide to Getting It On Again.* New York: Harper Collins. 2009.

Kerner I, Rinna L. *The Big, Fun, Sexy Sex Book.* New York: Gallery Books. 2012.

Kerner I. *She Comes First: The Thinking Man's Guide to Pleasuring a Woman.* New York: Regan Books. 2004.

Kingsley E. *Just Fuck Me! - What Women Want Men to Know About Taking Control in the Bedroom (A Guide for Couples).* Revised Ed. Secret Life Publishing: 2011.

Kerouac J. *On The Road.* New York: Viking. 1997.

Koskimäki J, Shiri R, Tammela T, Häkkinen J, Hakama M, Auvinen A. Regular intercourse protects against erectile dysfunction: Tampere Aging Male Urologic Study. *Am J Med.* 2008;121:592-6.

Lindenfors P, Tullberg BS. Evolutionary aspects of aggression: the importance of sexual selection. *Adv Genet.* 2011;75:7-22.

Little AC, Burriss RP, Petrie M, Jones BC, Roberts SC. Oral contraceptive use in women changes preferences for male facial masculinity and is associated with partner facial masculinity. *Psychoneuroendocrinology.* 2013;38:1777-85.

Litzinger S, Gordon KC. Exploring relationships among communication, sexual satisfaction, and marital satisfaction. *J Sex Marital Ther.* 2005;31:409-24.

Macdowall W, Gibson LJ, Tanton C, et al. Lifetime prevalence, associated factors, and circumstances of non-volitional sex in women and men in Britain: findings from the third National Survey of Sexual Attitudes and Lifestyles (Natsal-3). *Lancet.* 2013;382:1845-55.

Maclaran K, Panay N. Managing low sexual desire in women. *Womens Health (Lond Engl).* 2011;7:571-81.

Maio G, Saraeb S, Marchiori A. Physical activity and PDE5 inhibitors in the treatment of erectile dysfunction: results of a randomized controlled study. *J Sex Med.* 2010;7:2201-8.

Mansour RT, Aboulghar MA, Serour GI, Abbas AM, Ramzy AM, Rizk B. In vivo survival of spermatozoa in the human fallopian tube for 25 days: a case report. *J Assist Reprod Genet.* 1993;10:379-80.

Marchand E, Smolkowski K. Forced intercourse, individual and family context, and risky sexual behavior among adolescent girls. *J Adolesc Health.* 2013;52:89-95.

Marjoribanks J, Farquhar C, Roberts H, Lethaby A. Long term hormone therapy for perimenopausal and postmenopausal women. *Cochrane Database Syst Rev.* 2012 Jul 11;7:CD004143.

Mark KP, Janssen E, Milhausen RR. Infidelity in heterosexual couples: demographic, interpersonal, and personality-related predictors of extradyadic sex. *Arch Sex Behav.* 2011;40:971-82.

Mark KP, Murray SH. Gender differences in desire discrepancy as a predictor of sexual and relationship satisfaction in a college sample of heterosexual romantic relationships. *J Sex Marital* Ther. 2012;38:198-215.

Maserejian NN, Shifren J, Parish SJ, Segraves RT, Huang L, Rosen RC. Sexual arousal and lubrication problems in women with clinically diagnosed hypoactive sexual desire disorder: preliminary findings from the hypoactive sexual desire disorder registry for women. *J Sex Marital Ther.* 2012;38:41-62.

McBane SE, Borgelt LM, Barnes KN, Westberg SM, Lodise NM, Stassinos M. Use of compounded bioidentical hormone therapy in menopausal women: an opinion statement of the Women's Health Practice and Research Network of the American College of Clinical Pharmacy. *Pharmacotherapy.* 2014;34:410-23.

McMahon CG, Althof S, Waldinger MD, et al. An evidence-based definition of lifelong premature ejaculation: report of the International Society for Sexual Medicine (ISSM) ad hoc committee for the definition of premature ejaculation. BJU Int. 2008;102:338-50.

McNair P, Lewis G. Levels of evidence in medicine. *Int J Sports Phys Ther.* 2012;7:474-81.

Mehta D, Newport DJ, Frishman G, et al. Early predictive biomarkers for postpartum depression point to a role for estrogen receptor signaling. *Psychol Med.* 2014;5:1-14.

Menza TW, Kerani RP, Handsfield HH, Golden MR. Stable sexual risk behavior in a rapidly changing risk environment: findings from population-based surveys of men who have sex with men in Seattle, Washington, 2003-2006. *AIDS Behav.* 2011;15:319-29.

Milman LW, Sammel MD, Freeman E, Barnhart K, Dokras A. Higher serum testosterone levels correlate with increased risk of depressive symptoms in caucasian women through the entire menopausal transition. *Fertil Steril* 2013;100:S11.

Milne FH, Judge DS. A novel quantitative approach to women's reproductive strategies. PLoS One. 2012;7(10):e46760.

Monogamy. http://www.merriam-webster.com/dictionary/monogamy. Accessed September 4, 2014.

Morgentaler A. Testosterone, cardiovascular risk, and hormonophobia. *J Sex Med.* 2014;11:1362-6.

Mosbergen D. Cliteracy 101: Artist Sophia Wallace Wants You To Know The Truth About The Clitoris. Huffington Post. http://www.huffingtonpost.com/2013/08/28/cliteracy_n_3823983.html . August 29, 2013. Accessed August 10, 2014.

Muehlenhard CL, Shippee SK. Men's and women's reports of pretending orgasm. *J Sex Res.* 2010;47:552-567.

Mulhall J, King R, Glina S, Hvidsten K. Importance of and satisfaction with sex among men and women worldwide: results of the global better sex survey. *J Sex Med.* 2008;5:788-95.

Murray SH, Milhausen RR. Sexual desire and relationship duration in young men and women. *J Sex Marital Ther.* 2012;38:28-40.

Nastri CO, Lara LA, Ferriani RA, Rosa-E-Silva AC, Figueiredo JB, Martins WP. Hormone therapy for sexual function in perimenopausal and postmenopausal women. *Cochrane Database Syst Rev.* 2013 Jun 5;6:CD009672.

Nastri CO, Lara LA, Ferriani RA, Rosa-E-Silva AC, Figueiredo JB, Martins WP. Hormone therapy for sexual function in perimenopausal and postmenopausal women. *Cochrane Database Syst Rev.* 2013;6:CD009672.

National Vulvodynia Association. Fact Sheet. http://www.nva.org/fact_sheet.html . 2013. Accessed September 5, 2014.

Natland Fagerhaug T, Forsmo S, Jacobsen GW, Midthjell K, Andersen LF, Ivar Lund Nilsen T. A prospective population-based cohort study of lactation and cardiovascular disease mortality: the HUNT study. *BMC Public Health.* 2013;13:1070.

North American Menopause Society. The 2012 hormone therapy position statement of: The North American Menopause Society. *Menopause.* 2012;19:257-71.

Nunns D, Mandal D, Byrne M, et al; British Society for the Study of Vulval Disease (BSSVD) Guideline Group. Guidelines for the management of vulvodynia. *Br J Dermatol.* 2010; 162:1180-5.

Nurnberg HG, Hensley PL, Heiman JR, Croft HA, Debattista C, Paine S. Sildenafil treatment of women with antidepressant-associated sexual dysfunction: a randomized controlled trial. *JAMA.* 2008;300:395-404.

O'Connell HE, DeLancey JO. Clitoral anatomy in nulliparous, healthy, premenopausal volunteers using unenhanced magnetic resonance imaging. *J Urol.* 2005;173:2060-3.

O'Connell HE, Sanjeevan KV, Hutson JM. Anatomy of the clitoris. *J Urol.* 2005;174:1189-95.

Ondaatje M. *The English Patient: A Novel.* New York: Knopf. 1992.

Ott MA, Harezlak J, Ofner S, Fortenberry JD. Timing of incident STI relative to sex partner change in young women. *Sex Transm Dis.* 2012;39:747-9.

Panay N, Hamoda H, Arya R, Savvas M; British Menopause Society and Women's Health Concern. The 2013 British Menopause Society & Women's Health Concern recommendations on hormone replacement therapy. *Menopause Int.* 2013;19:59-68.

Paterson-Brown S. Should doctors reconstruct the vaginal introitus of adolescent girls to mimic the virginal state? Education about the hymen is needed. *BMJ.* 1998;316(7129).

Pazmany E, Bergeron S, Verhaeghe J, Van Oudenhove L, Enzlin P. Sexual communication, dyadic adjustment, and psychosexual well-being in premenopausal women with self-reported dyspareunia and their partners: a controlled study. *J Sex Med.* 2014;11:1786-97.

Pedersen AT, Iversen OE, Løkkegaard E, et al. Impact of recent studies on attitudes and use of hormone therapy among Scandinavian gynaecologists. *Acta Obstet Gynecol Scand.* 2007;86:1490-5

Peplau LA, Frederick DA, Yee C, Maisel N, Lever J, Ghavami N. Body image satisfaction in heterosexual, gay, and lesbian adults. *Arch Sex Behav.* 2009;38:713-25.

Perlis N, Lo KC, Grober ED, Spencer L, Jarvi K. Coital frequency and infertility: which male factors predict less frequent coitus among infertile couples? *Fertil Steril.* 2013;100:511-5.

Pitkin J. Should HRT be duration limited? *Menopause Int.* 2013;19:167-74.

Poels S, Bloemers J, van Rooij K, et al. Toward personalized sexual medicine (part 2): testosterone combined with a PDE5 inhibitor increases sexual satisfaction in women with HSDD and FSAD, and a low sensitive system for sexual cues. *J Sex Med.* 2013;10:810-23.

Porst H, Burnett A, Brock G, et al.; ISSM Standards Committee for Sexual Medicine. SOP conservative (medical and mechanical) treatment of erectile dysfunction. *J Sex Med.* 2013;10:130-71.

Practice Committee of American Society for Reproductive Medicine in collaboration with Society for Reproductive Endocrinology and Infertility. Optimizing natural fertility. *Fertil Steril.* 2008;90(5 Suppl):S1-6.

Pratt LA, Brody DJ, Gu Q. Antidepressant use in persons aged 12 and over: United States, 2005-2008. *NCHS Data Brief.* 2011;76:1-8.

Puppo V. La Sessualit_a Umana e l'educazione a Fare l'amore. Con Aggiornamenti. 2nd Ed. Florence, Italy. 2011.

Puppo V. Anatomia della vulva e del pene femminile: Clitoride-Piccole labbra-Bulbi del vestibolo-Uretra-Orgasmo femminile. Florence, Italy. 2014.

Puts DA, Dawood K, Welling LL. Why women have orgasms: an evolutionary analysis. *Arch Sex Behav.* 2012;41:1127-43.

Qin Z, Tian B, Wang X, Liu T, Bai J. Impact of frequency of intercourse on erectile dysfunction: a cross-sectional study in Wuhan, China. *J Huazhong Univ Sci Technolog Med Sci.* 2012;32:396-9.

Rebe KB, De Swardt G, Berman PA, Struthers H, McIntyre JA. Sexual lubricants in South Africa may potentially disrupt mucosal surfaces and increase HIV transmission risk among men who have sex with men. *S Afr Med J.* 2013;104:49-51.

Reece M, Herbenick D, Schick V, Sanders SA, Dodge B, Fortenberry JD. Sexual behaviors, relationships, and perceived health among adult men in the United States: results from a national probability sample. *J Sex Med.* 2010;7(Suppl 5):291-304.

Renfrew MJ, Craig D, Dyson L, McCormick F, Rice S, King SE, Misso K, Stenhouse E, Williams AF. Breastfeeding promotion for infants in neonatal units: a systematic review and economic analysis. Health Technol Assess. 2009;13:1-146.

Rhoden EL, Morgentaler A. Symptomatic response rates to testosterone therapy and the likelihood of completing 12 months of therapy in clinical practice. *J Sex Med.* 2010;7:277-83.

Richters J, de Visser RO, Rissel CE, Grulich AE, Smith AM. Demographic and psychosocial features of participants in bondage and discipline, "sadomasochism" or dominance and submission (BDSM): data from a national survey. *J Sex Med.* 2008;5:1660-8.

Roberts SC, Gosling LM, Carter V, Petrie M. MHC-correlated odour preferences in humans and the use of oral contraceptives. *Proc Biol Sci.* 2008;275:2715-22.

Roberts SC, Little AC, Burriss RP, et. al. Partner Choice, Relationship Satisfaction, and Oral Contraception: The Congruency Hypothesis. *Psychol Sci.* 2014;25:1497-1503.

Roney JR, Simmons ZL, Gray PB. Changes in estradiol predict within-women shifts in attraction to facial cues of men's testosterone. Psychoneuroendocrinology. 2011;36:742-9.

Rosenthal E. "A Push to Sell Testosterone Gels Troubles Doctors." The New York Times. http://www.nytimes.com/2013/10/16/us/a-push-to-sell-testosterone-gels-troubles-doctors.html?pagewanted=all&_r=0 . October 15, 2013. Accessed September 4, 2014.

Rosenwaks Z, Goldstien M, Fuerst ML. *A Baby at Last!: The Couple's Complete Guide to Getting Pregnant--from Cutting-Edge Treatments to Commonsense Wisdom.* New York, NY; Touchstone: 2010.

Rupp HA, James TW, Ketterson ED, Sengelaub DR, Ditzen B, Heiman JR. Lower sexual interest in postpartum women: relationship to amygdala activation and intranasal oxytocin. *Horm Behav.* 2013;63:114-21.

Sacco DF, Young SG, Brown CM, Bernstein MJ, Hugenberg K. Social exclusion and female mating behavior: rejected women show strategic enhancement of short-term mating interest. *Evol Psychol.* 2012;10:573-87.

Salmon C, Symons D. Slash fiction and human mating psychology. *J Sex Res.* 2004;41:94-100.

Sanchez DT, Moss-Racusin CA, Phelan JE, Crocker J. Relationship contingency and sexual motivation in women: implications for sexual satisfaction. *Arch Sex Behav.* 2011;40:99-110.

Santtila P, Wager I, Witting K, et al. Discrepancies between sexual desire and sexual activity: gender differences and associations with relationship satisfaction. *J Sex Marital* Ther. 2008;34:31-44.

Scarabin PY, Hemker HC, Clément C, Soisson V, Alhenc-Gelas M. Increased thrombin generation among postmenopausal women using hormone therapy: importance of the route of estrogen administration and progestogens. *Menopause*. 2011;18:873-9.

Scheele D, Striepens N, Güntürkün O, Deutschländer S, Maier W, Kendrick KM, Hurlemann R. Oxytocin modulates social distance between males and females. *J Neurosci*. 2012;32:16074-9.

Scheele D, Wille A, Kendrick KM, et al. Oxytocin enhances brain reward system responses in men viewing the face of their female partner. *Proc Natl Acad Sci USA*. 2013;110:20308-13.

Schooling CM, Au Yeung SL, Freeman G, Cowling BJ. The effect of statins on testosterone in men and women, a systematic review and meta-analysis of randomized controlled trials. *BMC Med*. 2013;11:57.

Seal BN, Meston CM. The impact of body awareness on sexual arousal in women with sexual dysfunction. *J Sex Med*. 2007;4:990-1000.

Setchell JM, Huchard E. The hidden benefits of sex: evidence for MHC-associated mate choice in primate societies. *Bioessays*. 2010;32:940-8.

Shah MB, Hoffstetter S. Contraception and sexuality. *Minerva Ginecol*. 2010;62:331-47.

Shindel AW, Nelson CJ, Naughton CK, Ohebshalom M, Mulhall JP. Sexual function and quality of life in the male partner of infertile couples: prevalence and correlates of dysfunction. *J Urol*. 2008;179:1056-9.

Shores MM, Moceri VM, Sloan KL, Matsumoto AM, Kivlahan DR. Low testosterone levels predict incident depressive illness in older men: effects of age and medical morbidity. *J Clin Psychiatry*. 2005;66:7-14.

Smith LJ, Mulhall JP, Deveci S, Monaghan N, Reid MC. Sex after seventy: a pilot study of sexual function in older persons. *J Sex Med*. 2007;4:1247-53.

Soares CN, Poitras JR, Prouty J. Effect of reproductive hormones and selective estrogen receptor modulators on mood during menopause. *Drugs Aging*. 2003;20:85-100.

Soares CN. Mood disorders in midlife women: understanding the critical window and its clinical implications. *Menopause*. 2014;21:198-206.

Somboonporn W, Davis S, Seif MW, Bell R. Testosterone for peri- and postmenopausal women. *Cochrane Database Syst Rev.* 2005 Oct 19;(4):CD004509.

Somers S. *I'm Too Young For This!* New York, NY: Harmony 2013

Somers S. *Sexy Forever: How to Fight Fat after Forty.* New York, NY: Harmony 2011.

Speroff L. Transdermal hormone therapy and the risk of stroke and venous thrombosis. *Climacteric.* 2010;13:429-32.

Sprecher S. Sexual satisfaction in premarital relationships: associations with satisfaction, love, commitment, and stability. *J Sex Res.* 2002;39:190-6.

Stephenson K, Neuenschwander PF, Kurdowska AK. The effects of compounded bioidentical transdermal hormone therapy on hemostatic, inflammatory, immune factors; cardiovascular biomarkers; quality-of-life measures; and health outcomes in perimenopausal and postmenopausal women. *Int J Pharm Compd.* 2013;17:74-85.

Stephenson KR, Ahrold TK, Meston CM. The association between sexual motives and sexual satisfaction: gender differences and categorical comparisons. *Arch Sex Behav.* 2011;40:607-18.

Stephenson KR, Meston CM. The young and the restless? Age as a moderator of the association between sexual desire and sexual distress in women. *J Sex Marital Ther.* 2012;38:445-57.

Stephenson KR, Meston CM. When are sexual difficulties distressing for women? The selective protective value of intimate relationships. *J Sex Med.* 2010;7:3683-94.

Stidham Hall K, Moreau C, Trussell J. Discouraging trends in reproductive health service use among adolescent and young adult women in the USA, 2002-2008. *Hum Reprod.* 2011;26:2541-8.

Studd J. Personal view: hormones and depression in women. *Climacteric.* 2014;21:1-3.

Studd JW. A guide to the treatment of depression in women by estrogens. *Climacteric.* 2011;14:637-42.

Tao P, Coates R, Maycock B. The impact of infertility on sexuality: A literature review. *Australas Med J.* 2011;4:620-7.

The Great Sperm Race. Dir. Julian Jones. Channel 4 Television Corporation, 2009. Television.

U.S. Department of Health & Human Services, Office of the Surgeon General. The Surgeon General's Call to Action to Support Breastfeeding [Fact Sheet]. http://www.surgeongeneral.gov/library/calls/breastfeeding/factsheet.html . 2014. Accessed September 5, 2014.

U.S. Department of Health & Human Services, Office on Women's Health. Sexual assault fact sheet. http://www.womenshealth.gov/publications/our-publications/fact-sheet/sexual-assault.html . July 16, 2012. Accessed September 4, 2014.

U.S. Food and Drug Administration. FDA evaluating risk of stroke, heart attack and death with FDA-approved testosterone products [Safety Announcement]. http://www.fda.gov/downloads/Drugs/DrugSafety/UCM383909.pdf . 2014. Accessed September 5, 2014.

U.S. Food and Drug Administration. Joint meeting for bone, reproductive and urologic drugs advisory committee and the drug safety and risk management advisory committee : FDA background documents for the discussion of two major issues in testosterone replacement therapy. http://www.fda.gov/downloads/AdvisoryCommittees/CommitteesMeetingMaterials/Drugs/ReproductiveHealthDrugsAdvisoryCommittee/UCM412536.pdf. September 17, 2014. Accessed September 24, 2014.

U.S. Food and Drug Administration. Menopause and Hormones: Common Questions [Consumer Information]. http://www.fda.gov/ForConsumers/ByAudience/ForWomen/ucm118624.htm#hormone_therapy_for_menopause . 2014. Accessed September 5, 2014.

Utian WH, Woods NF. Impact of hormone therapy on quality of life after menopause. *Menopause.* 2013;20:1098-105.

Utian WH. A decade post WHI, menopausal hormone therapy comes full circle--need for independent commission. *Climacteric.* 2012;15:320-5.

van Anders SM, Hipp LE, Kane Low L. Exploring co-parent experiences of sexuality in the first 3 months after birth. *J Sex Med.* 2013;10:1988-99.

Vigen R, O'Donnell CI, Barón AE, et al. Association of testosterone therapy with mortality, myocardial infarction, and stroke in men with low testosterone levels. *JAMA.* 2013;310:1829-36.

Virro MR, Larson-Cook KL, Evenson DP. Sperm chromatin structure assay (SCSA) parameters are related to fertilization, blastocyst development, and ongoing pregnancy in in vitro fertilization and intracytoplasmic sperm injection cycles. *Fertil Steril.* 2004;81:1289-95.

Wade LD, Kremer EC, Brown J. The incidental orgasm: the presence of clitoral knowledge and the absence of orgasm for women. *Women Health.* 2005;42:117-38.

Wallace S. CLITERACY, 100 Natural Laws. http://www.sophiawallace.com/cliteracy-100-natural-laws . 2012. Accessed September 10, 2014.

Weiss P, Brody S. Women's partnered orgasm consistency is associated with greater duration of penile-vaginal intercourse but not of foreplay. *J Sex Med.* 2009;6:135-41.

Weschler T. *Taking Charge of Your Fertility: The Definitive Guide to Natural Birth Control, Pregnancy Achievement, and Reproductive Health* (Rev. ed.). New York, NY: Collins. 2006.

Weschler T. *Cycle Savvy: The Smart Teen's Guide to the Mysteries of Her Body.* New York: Collins, 2006.

Whisman MA, Gordon KC, Chatav Y. Predicting sexual infidelity in a population-based sample of married individuals. *J Fam Psychol.* 2007;21:320-4.

Wilcox, W. The State of Our Unions. http://www.stateofourunions.org/index.php . December 16, 2012. Accessed June 5, 2014.

Wilkinson TA, Vargas G, Fahey N, Suther E, Silverstein M. "I'll see what I can do": What adolescents experience when requesting emergency contraception. *J Adolesc Health.* 2014;54:14-9.

Willoughby BJ, Farero AM, Busby DM. Exploring the effects of sexual desire discrepancy among married couples. *Arch Sex Behav.* 2014;43:551-62.

Willoughby BJ, Vitas J. Sexual desire discrepancy: the effect of individual differences in desired and actual sexual frequency on dating couples. *Arch Sex Behav.* 2012;4:477-86.

Wismeijer AA, van Assen MA. Psychological characteristics of BDSM practitioners. *J Sex Med.* 2013;10:1943-52.

Woods NF, Mitchell ES, Smith-Di Julio K. Sexual desire during the menopausal transition and early postmenopause: observations from the Seattle Midlife Women's Health Study. *J Womens Health (Larchmt).* 2010;19:209-18.

World Health Organization. *WHO Laboratory Manual for the Examination of Human Semen and Sperm-Cervical Mucus Interaction,* 4th edition. Cambridge University Press, Cambridge. 1999.

Wright RW Jr, Anderson GB, Cupps PT, Drost M. Successful culture in vitro of bovine embryos to the blastocyst stage. *Biol Reprod.* 1976;14:157-62.

Yassin AA, Saad F. Testosterone and erectile dysfunction. *J Androl.* 2008;29:593-604.

Ziller V, Heilmaier C, Kostev K. Time to pregnancy in subfertile women in German gynecological practices: analysis of a representative cohort of more than 60,000 patients. *Arch Gynecol Obstet.* 2014 Sep 4. [Epub ahead of print].

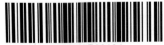

Made in the USA
San Bernardino, CA
11 November 2014